The Ugly Side of Hope

A Journey Through Infertility

LUANNE ROSE

The Ugly Side of Hope

A Journey Through Infertility

©2022 Luanne Rose

print ISBN: 978-1-66786-176-0
ebook ISBN: 978-1-66786-177-7

About the Author:

Why does this feel like I am filling out yet another online dating profile? Thought I was past this. Hi, I'm Luanne. I'm kind dorky and extremely sarcastic. Despite this I still manage to have great friends, two cute dogs and an amazing guy who loves all of me. I am super obsessed with all things Disney and randomly collect owls. (It's a whole story.) I like to quilt but am not amazing at it. I have been writing about myself with hopes to publish since a young age. I remember once typing out all my journal entries with the idea of giving it to friends to read in the 5th grade. Ironically most people reading this are those same 5th grade people. I hope you enjoy.

Dedication:

It was impossible for me to decide who to choose to dedicate this book to. So, I dedicate this book to Suzi. I was first inspired to write this book after finding an old note from her: "Earth life gives us challenges. The Lord gives us the ability to turn those trials into helping others, He has blessed you with the knowledge and the power to bless the lives of others who you can now understand. You are here to do great things." I also dedicate this book to Mike. He was the first one to read it. Beyond that he was in my corner in ways I needed him to be at times I needed it the most. His love and support of me is beyond comprehension. Thank you, Mom and Dad Hardy, for loving me as one of your own. That love and support was exactly what I needed in order to get my story out. I love you both and miss you always.

Special Thanks:

Thank you to Lyssa for taking the time and energy to edit and give amazing feedback. Thank you to my husband, Robert, for supporting me through the final days of getting this done. Thank you to Toni & Chelsey for not only being there for me through a lot of the actual things that happened to me but through the writing process and the help in the naming of the book. Thank you to my mom, Trish and Amanda for providing feedback to help me get my book to where it needed to be. Finally, thank you to all the others who listened to me cry and cheered me on every step of the way.

Preface

There are several different events in your life that you never forget. Your graduation day. Your first kiss. The first day at your first job. Your wedding day. You get it. These are days that stay burned into your mind, waiting as reminders of different emotions in your life. Most people have these same days in their lives. The joys are shared with "tweets" and on social media in various Instagram and Facebook posts. We are all quick to show the happiness of it all.

I love looking back at special moments. I love the happiness they bring and the smile that creeps across my face as I soak in the memories. I have a lot of these memories, and I remember every detail of them. Between all the joys, though, I do have one memory that has defined me more than any other. A dark one that pours sadness and heartache into my life, unlike the happy moments. The memory was made on a day I will never forget.

I had an appointment at 7:00 AM. I remember feeling grateful that I had the work-life and scheduling flexibility I had so I could make all of the appointments. My last appointment had not been that great. The doctor said I was "progressing slowly" but, "not all hope was lost." We would go a few more days, and then we would decide if I was done trying.

For the two weeks leading up to my appointment, I had spent hours obsessively injecting medication into my body. As a diabetic the injections were not strange to me. But the mixing of medicines and the amounts; even the preciseness of it all was new. My fridge was packed with medications and I wasn't even sure what they did.

In addition to the medication regimen, I had to get my blood drawn every other day. I would arrive at 7:00 AM and I couldn't eat beforehand. I also had to go to various doctor appointments so other specialists could check the progress as well.

This particular appointment that stings my memory was on a Saturday. Since it was the weekend, I was the only one there. It was dark. The Physician's Assistant only had the lights on in the room we were using, so everything else faded away. The nurse brought me into the small room, and I prepared for my exam, which included disrobing. I laid on the cold table, breathing. Waiting. Wondering. After what seemed like the longest stretch of time the PA walked in and completed the exam. She said things were "not promising" and in fact that what we were afraid of had happened. She told me to get dressed and meet her in the office next door. I sat up, took a deep breath and told myself to be strong. I wasn't sure if I was strong as I put my clothes back on. I had no idea what she was going to say or what my options would be. I just continued my inner dialogue and told myself this moment wouldn't define me. I was very wrong. After a deep breath I went to the next room over and I sat down at the desk that the PA was already waiting for me and she began to tell me a few things.

The amount of medication I had been taking was the absolute max they recommended giving patients.

I had taken the medication for the longest time they could give it to take effect on my body.

Then… then she said they had discovered that only one follicle, or egg, had formed. Even though it only takes one egg, the egg was not in good "health," and the likelihood of it doing the job it was supposed to do was small. She said I had a less than 5% chance of having children of my own.

I don't know if my brain just needed time to process this or if I was denying my body the ability to react. Either way I just sat and stared at her, past her, as she delivered the news. She pushed a box of tissues my way and asked if I had any questions. I went to open my mouth to ask about options and instead started to cry. As if reading my mind, she did start to tell me my options. It was either egg donation IVF, bringing my odds of having a child to 60%, or adoption, which would make my odds of having a child 100%. She said that my insurance would not cover egg donation IVF because of the legal issues that come with this type of fertility treatment. This meant either way, the road ahead was expensive and hard, and I had some choices to make. After our conversation, I got in my car and drove numbly to work.

At the time, I was an Assistant Manager for a well-known bakery and café chain. As a woman in charge, I didn't believe in letting my team see me cry. It felt like a weakness that I wasn't able to show. During the 30 minute commute from Point Loma to Mira Mesa, I did everything I could to pull myself together, but nothing seemed to work.

By the time I arrived, I had managed to stop crying long enough to go inside the café and grab the shift supervisor and shove her into the office. I sat her in the chair and stood in front of the window so no one could see in. I started to tell her what happened and began to sob uncontrollably. She got up and hugged me. Tight. Told me she was sorry and told me to go home. So that's what I did. I drove home, sat on my bed and cried. I felt so defeated and ... I don't know, broken. Lost. Alone. I had a friend who was going through the same fertility treatment I had just been defeated by. I sent her a text message and told her what was happening. She offered words of comfort, and even though it was sweet, it didn't do anything.

Over the next few days and weeks and months, I started to feel better and feel like I could have a future as a mother. However, even though the wound seemed to heal, the reality was it wasn't healing at all. Infertility is not something you "get over." It's not something you get past and move on from. It's not something that heals. It is something you learn to manage over time. It's like a tree that is covered in vines. The vines cling to the tree and take the tree's water and sunlight. Its livelihood. Even though all of this is stolen from the tree, the tree still lives. It still grows. It finds a way. The same is true with infertility. It takes your energy and your livelihood, but you still live. You still grow. You still find a way.

I am infertile. This is my story.

Chapter 1

When people find out I am infertile the same things seem to happen. First, I can tell they feel uncomfortable; it's in the face. Then, they say they are sorry. Then, because they don't know what to do or say and I think it is human nature to try to make people feel better, they say one of following:

Oh well, you can just adopt, right?

Aren't you young? You have plenty of time.

Well, some people never have kids, and they are happy.

You can come watch my kids. They are monsters and will make you feel grateful.

My sister's friend's aunt couldn't have kids, but then when she tried <insert some diet or yoga practice here> and got pregnant instantly.

You need to relax. Once you relax, it will happen.

Finally, the subject changes quickly, and they move on.

I am guessing that this scenario feels familiar to you. Most likely, you have been on one end of this conversation. Maybe you are the uncomfortable friend, family member or neighbor just trying to get past a subject that you know nothing about. You don't realize the hurt it's causing the person on the other side of the conversation, and you don't know it is much more complicated than the short, easy answers you just gave. Even if you do, you don't know what to say to make it okay. Perhaps you are the woman on the other side who hears one of these things and politely nods, while inside your tears, anger and fear are being pushed down.

Before I go any further, I want to explain something. If you are the person that is uncomfortable and unsure of what to say, I can speak for the infertile community. We know that your intentions are not to be hurtful. For the most part, I can say that I am sure you are sincerely just trying to say to the person "Don't feel defeated, have hope, I'm sorry." But, next time you ask someone if they have children or want children and they say, "Oh I am infertile," even if you know little about them or the situation, a simple "I'm sorry" is all they need. Honestly. Even from a stranger, the words "I'm sorry" go a long way. They will let you know if they want to talk about it further and what direction they want to go. Just be open and willing to listen to the struggles they face.

Very recently, I was at a work conference. During a lunch break, I sat down at a table with a new guy on my team. We all work from home and travel a lot, so it's not often you can welcome a new team member face to face and learn about them in the beginning. As we sat and chatted, he commented on my many tattoos. Asked if I was a punk rocker or a tough chick. I laughed and said I just liked tattoos. He pointed, as a lot of people do, to the elephant that is on my right forearm. This tattoo has an adult elephant that is drawn out in fine lines. Behind the elephant are splashes of watercolor in baby blue and pink. Then, coming out of the elephant's trunk is the word "hope." It's a beautiful tattoo and not at all small so it can be seen easily. He said it was really pretty and loved the detail and work. I thanked him for his compliment and explained the meaning behind it. I told him that it was an infertility tattoo. I said that I couldn't have kids, so it's a reminder for me not to give up hope. He fell right into the same mold of telling me that I could adopt and encouraged me not to say I can't have kids because I can.

For the most part, I can smile and nod to any subject, even if it is hurtful. I usually know that hurting me is not the intention and can move past it. However, every once in a while, the comment cuts deeper than usual. It happens when I'm tired or caught off guard. That day was both. I was tired and the comment caught me off guard because I was being commanded not to be upset and acknowledge that kids could come in my life. I politely responded that adoption was not as easy as it sounds. He said he understood. Then said he didn't know my belief, but Sarah, from the Bible, couldn't have a baby and look at what happened to her. At this point, my brain caught up with my mouth. I was able to take a deep breath and not give the first response that came to me, which was definitely not the best. Instead, I nodded and smiled. I calmly explained that there is a difference between adoption and giving birth and said I appreciated his thoughts.

I found myself upset at him. I found his comments rude. All I could think about was the trials and heartaches over the past (at this point) ten years I've had that got me to the point of comprehending and accepting that I can't have my own children. I thought about my experience with adoption and the insane number of tears I have cried over this invisible disease I have. However, he couldn't see or possibly know any. He had no idea, no experience in the world of infertility. How could I hold him to this standard of expectations to respond the right way? That being said, why should I have to deal with the suggestions that are so gut-wrenching I can sometimes barely comprehend my answers?

A few years ago, I decided to become very vocal about my infertility. I became not at all afraid to express my struggles and thoughts and feelings that come with it. I have written blogs, Facebook posts and shared Instagram pictures expressing my emotions surrounding infertility. Some people are private, and rightfully so, about their infertility. Some people don't even tell their parents. But I have not been shy and share every chance I get. I decided that while so many people are giving inappropriate responses to "I am infertile," I could take advantage of my ability to proclaim and share my experiences to educate. I realized that with education comes understanding, and if I took the time to share why the simple answers bullet-pointed above are not answers at all, the answers might stop. I don't expect someone who is not infertile to fully understand what an infertile person is going through. However, I hope by reading this, you can understand a sliver of what the infertile woman in your life is suffering through and can gain a better grasp on why the words "I'm sorry" and listening is all that is needed.

In this book, I will be sharing my experiences and my experiences alone. I can not speak for every infertile woman on every subject. Even though we share heartache, we are still individuals that go through this experience differently. It doesn't matter how different the path is, though. We are all getting through and just trying to hang on to hope.

I would like to also add that I wrote this book over many years, and my life has changed while writing this book. My view on religion has changed. I have changed partners and where I lived. That being said, my experiences stand the same. These experiences have still shaped me and helped me become me. For what would be life without change and experience?

Chapter 2

Thinking about not bearing my own children is devastating. Despite the fact that a PA told me in an office, complete with facts and figures, that I will most likely not have my own doesn't mean I accepted it then. In fact that was just a small moment in what has felt like a lifetime of accepting that my body doesn't work the way I expected it to — that everything from my childhood leading to adulthood included having children and all expectations related to it are not possible. As I have worked through and come to understand my struggles with infertility, I had to first realize why I even wanted kids to begin with. So, I took some time to look back on my life.

As you become an adult and start thinking about your future, you start making decisions such as your career path, whether or not to get married and what your family life will look like. Based on your life experiences, sometimes without even realizing it, you start to steer your life in the direction of however you answer these questions. For me I felt like these three, kind of four specific questions were answered for me. I never really remember thinking about them. I just remember that my life was to go in one direction. I would go to college, get married, start a family and become a stay at home mom. It was so clear and set in stone.

I was one of those little girls who always had a baby doll growing up. I remember I loved to play house. I would play Mom all the time. I loved to change my baby's diapers and feed them. I would do their hair, give them names and put them to bed. My parents got me some pretty cool toys and a couple of them were beyond amazing. One was a high-chair that hooked to your dining room table where a baby could fit. The other was a car seat that actually fit in the car and held your baby. If it was just me and my mom or my dad, I could hook up the baby in the car seat while we rode in the car. Man, I loved playing Mom.

As I grew up, I soon realized that even though I loved playing Mom, I did not have that maternal instinct I noticed most women had. I hated babysitting. Well, unless it was the type of babysitting where the kids are asleep the whole time, so you get to watch TV and eat the food in the fridge. I would seriously loved those gigs. I would go to the house and get the kids in bed as soon as I could. I'm sure they all went to bed before their bedtime every night I was there. That made me a good sitter, right? Right. Beyond this, I was never one to look at a baby and think, "Oh! How cute and perfect I want one." I would say that out loud because I didn't want the world to think I was a weirdo, but I didn't feel it. Also, kids younger than me were never my thing. I didn't really want to be around them or play with them. I didn't want anything to do with them. This seemed opposite to all of my other friends.

In my senior year, I did that class in high school where you get a "baby" for a few days. The type that records how well you take care of it. Worst three days of my life. I didn't think it was fun for one minute. I wanted to be out with my friends having fun. Not attached to an anchor that cried. Still, as I think about that baby and knowing what my life was like, I cringe remembering how unattached I was to that thing. I did enjoy scrapbooking my experience, though. I think I can safely say I turned in one of the most decorative reports on having a baby ever in the history of that class.

Chapter 3

Even though I wasn't very motherly, becoming a mother and having a family was just something that I expected to happen, and it seemed to be expected of me. I grew up in a church where the focus on family was really big. In my classes as a kid, we would sing songs about families and moms and dads. We would learn stories and were taught that having a family was important. As I got older, we learned as young women what it took to become a great mother. What we had to do then to reach the goal of growing up right and starting a family. Being a strong role model for your children and bringing up the house in righteousness. Even though I don't disagree with the idea of growing up to become a mom, those teachings at such a young age affect you at your core. They feel like sitting in front of a TV screen with your eyelids forced open as the words "become a mom" scrolls for hours — like my only true worth in life was in becoming a mother.

Not only did my church seem to have an agenda of opening me to the eyes of motherhood, but my community did too. I grew up in a small town. The popular thing was to have five or more kids, and most siblings were very close in age. Buying groceries in bulk and large cars seemed to be the most popular trend. I sometimes felt it was like a contest to see who could have the most kids and how close to 9 months in age could you get them to be. There weren't really any small families. In fact, I only knew of one friend who was an only child.

Another obvious influence in my life that made me want to be a mom was my own family. I like to think we were a pretty normal family. Up until my freshman year of high school, my parents were married, and they raised me, my older sister, and my younger sister. The older sister, Valerie, is three years older than me and we were...how do you say...classic in our love for each other as sisters. Valerie got to spend three glorious years as the only child. I'm sure she was waited on hand and foot and my parents just adored her. Naturally, you can understand her initial distaste for me when I finally did join the family. I don't remember her level of non-appreciation when we were young, but one time she was helping me down the stairs and I fell and dislocated my shoulder. Rumor has it that she pushed me. Imagine the fun that must have been for my parents. This is after a mistake of a certain parent *coughs* dad *coughs* who dropped me and I broke my leg. Yes, you are thinking correctly, social services did visit my house. The drama between me and my older sister did not stop there. In the 15 years we lived together we fought more than we got along. I always just wanted to get along with Valerie and she was often "too cool" for me. That being said, every once in a blue moon a friendship would appear consisting of making up dance routines, recitals, plays and playing video games. Beyond that, though, it was loud yelling, knife throwing, punching, screaming and general "Now that you are in high school, Luanne, do not even think about coming over to my table and talking to my friends" type situations. Everyone promised me that Valerie and I would get along once she moved out but I never saw that day coming. They were right, though. We are now friends and laugh about how I used to torture her with the song "Sombrero Sam" on the piano and she would do whatever she could to make sure I knew I was loved less by everyone in the family. Ah yes, Valerie.

I have a much different relationship with my younger sister, Frankie, for many reasons. Frankie is 5 years younger than me. I never felt jealous of her. I actually remember the very first time I saw her. She was a new baby at the hospital with my mom. My mom and dad let me hold her. She was so little and cute. She has always stayed little and cute. Frankie kind of got the short end of the stick in the family. She had to be little and deal with the stress of a divorce and broken family at a young and developmental age. No one was there to look out for her, so she had to look out for herself. It has made her independent, which is good, but it also meant that my relationship didn't really develop with her until we were both older. She was always my sister and I always loved her with everything I had, but I didn't always know her and who she was. She was just the cute little girl who, when not dressed up in boy clothes, walked around naked and did whatever she could to not wear a dress. A few years ago she came out as bisexual. This was a big moment for her. So, I had to hold back my laughter as I thought to myself, I know Frank...I know.

My dad could do anything. Even though he had a full-time job, he fixed cars, built stuff out of wood (he totally finished our unfinished basement by himself) and cooked. He was also a pretty avid runner. Later in my life I developed this same love of running. I then soon discovered we not only have the same heart for running, but the same feet, and we both had to have the same total foot reconstruction surgery on our right feet so we could run again. Not fun. Growing up, he would travel for work. When he traveled, he would think of us, never returning home without a small gift. One time he brought home a coloring book and crayons that had sparkles in them. Crayons with sparkles! I still think about those crayons and how happy they made me. He also took us to travel with him. Craziest thing I will ever say is my best memories with my dad lie at Battle Mountain, NV. If you are Valerie, right now you are agreeing. If you are literally any other human being on the planet, you are wondering what is so great about the armpit of Nevada. Besides a super amazing Mexican restaurant...nothing. It's just where my dad took me once to spend time with just him and his work and I loved it.

My mom stayed at home most of the time. She bounced from working to being at home to working from home. She sold Avon, Tupperware, lingerie. And she worked as a dental assistant, front desk receptionist, and lastly, as a cosmetologist. When she was home, my mom would cook, clean and take care of the house. She would sew our dance costumes, Christmas pajamas, Halloween costumes and who knows what else. She was always innovative in the way she would get us to do our chores and literally sang about everything. It was actually a running joke that she could figure out a song to go with everything. For the record, I also have this skill.

I was always amazed by both of my parents. They did everything in our house. Furniture was made by them. Meals were always cooked from scratch. It especially amazes me now that I am an adult. Do you know how I make taco meat? I buy the packet of taco seasoning from the store and pour it over meat. I even went to culinary school and this is how I make tacos. My parents had their own recipe of mixed ingredients they used! I think for the rest of my life, I am going to be trying to make food as good as my parents (and will never succeed). In addition they always tried really hard to create good memories. Christmas, ski trips, family vacations, camping... you name it and we did it. Even though it was far from perfect, it was a great world to grow up in.

We were one of the smaller families in my hometown. I have to say we were pretty impressed that we could all fit in one "normal sized" car. My dad once told me, I think as a joke, that having three or less kids was the best because it meant that when we went on vacation we could rent the cheapest car. I mean...he's not wrong. Growing up in my family, just like any family, had its ups and downs. Even though both good and bad memories firmly build the foundation we live our life on, I think that for the most part, we remember the best part of our childhoods. Weed out a lot of the bad. I know I did. I do remember a lot of the shit that I went through as a kid, but I cherish the good memories. So many stand out to me. For one, we had some pretty awesome traditions growing up. One of my favorites was our family breakfast. Most families have goals of having dinner together but my parents realized that this was a pretty unrealistic goal for us. Between work, friends, dance practice and other activities it was very rare that we would even see each other at night, let alone eat together. So, instead, we had breakfast almost every morning together. My parents would wake us up earlier than normal, so we could eat and clean up before leaving for school and work. Most mornings, we had a huge breakfast planned for us. Sometimes it was an assortment of cereals on the table, but that was rare. And during our meal, we would talk about what was ahead for the day and the things we had planned. It's easy to see why this was an amazing tradition. It guaranteed a meal together and started our days out right.

It's funny to look back on this memory. Just like I mentioned before, we tend to weed out the shit. As I look back, like really look back, I am able to glimpse two very upset girls (my older sister and I) not wanting to get out of bed at 7:00 AM when they knew good and well that a simple skip of our family tradition would mean at least a half-hour more of sleep. Even thinking of that, though, it still brings a smile to my face. I love that my parents fought through the whining and the tears and the frustrations. They did that and gained family experiences we cherish forever.

Another great tradition was the way we celebrated birthdays. It was a week-long event at our house. One night in the week we would go out to eat as a family and whoever's birthday it was got to decide what restaurant we went to. We had a friend party, a family party (this included the aunts and uncles and cousins) and one night we got to decide what we were having for dinner, and we got to eat it on the red plate. That's right; we had a special red plate. I have no idea how this tradition got started. I don't even know where that red plate came from. What I do know is every year you looked forward to that red plate meal. Not only did I enjoy eating off the red plate, but I enjoyed setting the table and having the red plate out for someone else. It was something so small that meant so much.

My all-time favorite traditions and favorite childhood memories come from the Fourth of July. In fact, these memories are so great that, to this day, I can't seem to find a way to enjoy the Fourth I am very often left feeling like the day was a big letdown. What made it so great? First, I should mention that my mom is an amazing seamstress. If I can sew half as good as my mom one day, I will have accomplished a lot in my life. She had a room in the house that was just her sewing room. It had a huge cutting table, a closet full of fabric, and two beautiful machines. One year, my mom made my sisters and I some shirts out of flag fabric. We also made scrunchies to match. Later, we found shoes that were made out of the same fabric! They were a must buy. My older sister and I would wear three pairs of socks every year on the 4th; one red pair, one pair white and one blue pair. Layered, of course. It may have been 100 degrees, but it was worth it because with the whole outfit together, we looked nothing short of fabulous. Our Fourth always involved us getting up super early in the morning and dragging camping chairs down to the parade route. At the parade, they would hand out little flags for us to wave and candy to collect. Needless to say, it was pretty much every child's dream.

After the parade, we would go to a friend's BBQ, a baseball game or head home. I'm sure my parents napped while my sister and I played in the afternoon and got ready for the night. A few hours before sundown, we would gather up food, games, the grill and our Fourth of July blanket. We would pile into the car and head to the river.

I don't care what anyone says about it; my hometown has always had the best fireworks in the world. It seemed like the whole town would go down to the river to wait for a spectacular show, knowing it would be better each year we went. While we waited for the sun to go down, we would grill burgers, play games and walk around to see if we could find anyone we knew. Then, as soon as it got dark, we would turn our radios up and wait. Everyone would stare into the sky as firework after firework exploded, synchronized with the music. Just thinking of it now makes me well up a little bit. The show was never short of amazing.

Then, even though my parents were tired and had just driven through insane traffic, we would go home and light off our own fireworks. It was never anything fancy, but it was always fun. Every Fourth growing up ended with a feeling of love in my heart for the members of my family. The love for them and my country always took over my thoughts as I laid in bed and relived the day.

In addition to cool holiday traditions, we traveled a lot growing up. My dad's family lived in Southern California, so we would visit there about once a year — and sometimes my parents would put just the kids on a plane so we could visit Oma and Opa by ourselves. We also took ski trips throughout the year, including one longer stay at a big ski resort. Another family favorite was camping. My parents really rocked at camping. We had tents, amazing food and fun games and activities planned. I loved roasting marshmallows, swimming and fishing.

One year my parents either really saved up or went into insane debt and took us to Disney World. Best. Vacation. Ever. It was the only vacation on record where my older sister and I didn't fight. It is also logged as the vacation where I got the worst sunburn I have ever had. Thank you Florida.

Even though I could probably write about a thousand pages on my family traditions and how great they were, I will move on. Growing up was pretty normal for us, and my parents were hands-on.

It was obvious that my parents didn't want a large family. Nothing wrong with that. The three of us were just so perfect they didn't need more. Or we were so horrible… Either way, like I had said before, we were pretty excited that we all fit in a normal size car. I can't speak for my younger sister since we never really played together due to our age difference, but my older sister and I used to play "house" and "babies" all the time - me more than her. My mom would always humor me by asking my baby's name and calling herself grandma. She would let me hold it and cradle it like it was my own and encourage me to hone in on these motherly skills that I once had. We talked about having kids when I grew up, and she'd often say, "Just wait, when you have children, they will be twice as bad as you," the ultimate mother's curse. One time I asked my mom when I would be allowed to swear in front of her, and she said when I have kids of my own. Both of my parents often made comments like, "when you have a family," or "when you have kids." There was never pressure to have kids and a family, but it just seemed like it was expected. Like it was the normal thing to do.

That's the thing. I can't seem to pinpoint a single event that made me want to have kids or made me expect to have kids. I think it was just simply being surrounded by a community and church that was focused on families. By being involved in amazing traditions and growing up in a home where family was important, I just always expected to have one of my own. I can't think of a time in my childhood where I ever thought that maybe I wouldn't have a family. I can even look back at the TV I watched, like Roseanne, and recognize its influence on my psyche. The show was about her, not about her sister, who wasn't married and didn't have kids. We also had "Family Matters" and "Full House." Families. Everywhere.

I can't think of a time in my life where I believed not having a family was even possible. The first glimpse of this was with a cousin of mine. As I mentioned, my dad's family lived in California, and we would always make it a point to go and visit everyone. My dad is ten years younger than his older sibling, who is closest in age. So, my cousins were older than me. They always loved me and always made me feel like I was important in their lives, but they were older. I had two cousins get married close to the same time. I don't remember who got married first, but I remember attending both wedding receptions. And as society teaches us, once there is marriage next comes babies.

One year while visiting family, we were at one of my cousin's houses, one of the newly married ones. I must have been between eight and ten years old. I don't remember all the details, but I remember one cousin was pregnant, and one cousin, the one who's house we were at, was not. My mom and this not yet pregnant cousin were talking about it in the kitchen when she started to cry. My mom wrapped her arms around her, and they walked into a room and shut the door. They were in there for a while.

I later asked my mom what had happened. She said that this cousin was sad about her sister-in-law being pregnant. I asked why she would be sad. My mom said that sometimes when you want a baby, and someone else gets one first, it can be sad. That memory stuck with me. My cousin did have a baby. In fact, she was blessed with three beautiful children who are all amazing and a perfect combination of her and her husband.

This was it though. This is the only instance I remember where the possibility that there couldn't be a family in my future was even a thought. That having kids might not come naturally. It's such a fuzzy memory that I am not even sure if it counts. Even with this memory the thought of not being able to have a family never crossed my mind.

Over the years, through different interactions with different people, I have learned and come to really understand that we are a product of the environment we grew up in. That doesn't mean we don't become individuals with our own beliefs, ideas and life. But inherently, we believe that dads do car things if your dad was the only one who worked on the car. Maybe we believe moms do the baking because your mom made cinnamon rolls for every member of the church for Christmas, yes every single member, because making cinnamon rolls is what she liked to do. Is there anything wrong with that? No. Maybe your dad just really liked working on cars, and your mom would rather focus on baking. It might be cliché, but it's also true. There is nothing wrong with it. However, it's the environment you grew up in, and so your ideas and thoughts and expectations grow with you.

Chapter 4

There was nothing wrong with the environment I grew up in. I do have my opinions on some things, but for the most part, there is not much I would change. A focus on families and children and traditions is great. Celebrated even. I wouldn't want to grow up without a focus on family. It seems like perhaps I should write a "but…" and yet there isn't one. I just want to paint a picture as to why I want a family and why I feel empty that I don't have one. Why it's not an easy idea to let go of no matter the circumstances. There are parts of you that you can't let go of. I don't think it's fair to tell me that some people are happy without kids, so I might end up ok too. Because you're asking me to change who I am. Who I want to be. Who I grew up believing I was.

My years of dealing with infertility have been brutal. As you read my story and hear my struggles and heartaches and all the tries to become a mother, you might realize how much I am unable then and now to give up on becoming a mom. You will see I am unable to give up on having the future life I created in my mind. This image created just by the act of simply growing up.

I was a teenager when I realized that, in between my feelings of not always liking kids or lacking a motherly instinct and experiencing the positives of having family around me, I really did want my own. I wanted a big family. Lots of kids and tons of memories and traditions to share. I shared this desire with my friends, and we would dream about it together. I even had a friend who would stay up late with me to pick out our future children's names and give them ridiculous spellings. Of course, they all had the last name of our current crush, like typical teenagers. We all wanted to be moms one day.

The reality of motherhood was introduced to me at the age of fifteen. Up until this point, becoming a mom seemed like a fantasy for the future. Then one of my friends from high school got pregnant. I eventually had several friends get pregnant in high school, plus a handful of people I knew but wasn't friends with and all but one of them kept their babies. The first one got married soon after the baby was born and was forced to grow up fast. Her wedding was very weird because I felt separated from it all. It was like being in a dream. We were both sixteen. Her husband was seventeen. They lived in her room at her parent's house, and for a while, I lost touch with her. Her life quickly became drastically different than mine. I was trying to get my first kiss and first real boyfriend. She was taking care of a baby and had a husband.

A few years after she got married and had a second child, a mutual friend of ours found out that she was in a little trouble. Her marriage was, understandably, falling apart, and they couldn't make ends meet. This mutual friend and I got together and went grocery shopping for her. We broke into her apartment and filled her fridge. Then when she got home, we sat and talked with her. I remember thinking how sorry I felt for her. I just wanted to hug her. I couldn't imagine being that young and having two kids and my own apartment. A husband that was really still a boy. Each of them growing up while expected by others to be grown up. Even though the state of my life wasn't fantastic, it made me grateful I still had time to be a teenager.

One of my friends who got pregnant was a year older than me. I interacted with her the most during her pregnancy. She moved into a small apartment with her boyfriend. And I remember thinking it was so cool that she got to have her own place. They would both stay up late and work and buy what they wanted at the grocery store. They even had their own TV. It was so awesome. I spent a lot of time there since I was friends with both of them. I remember she had decorated their room really cute. She hung up both of their personalized parking spot signs from their senior year of high school on the wall. It's funny how something that seemed so cool and grown-up then now seems really juvenile. We always had fun at their house, though.

Then the baby came. I remember the very first time I went over to their house after he was born. It was also one of my last visits. While I was there, my friend fed the baby, bathed the baby and then got him dressed. During these activities, I was trying to talk to her about my most recent boy problems and friend problems and she didn't really seem interested. At one point, she laid him on his changing table, naked, in preparation of getting him ready. She had to grab something from the bathroom and asked me to make sure he didn't roll out. I just stared at him. He started to cry, and that turned into a scream. I literally had no idea what to do. He just screamed and screamed and there I was, waiting for my friend to come back. She finally came back and side-eyed me and sighed and picked him up to comfort him. I suddenly felt very out of place. I realized this was now my friend's world, and I was no longer a part of it. I didn't feel wanted and honestly, I didn't want to be there. I wanted to worry about the tattoo I was getting that night and whose house I was going to party at. I didn't want this grown-up life.

I stayed in touch with my friend because I loved her and had loved spending time with her. We just didn't hang out as much. I remember finding out that she got engaged, which felt like a mistake to me but also wasn't my place to say anything. Sometime after getting engaged, they decided instead to break it off. I went over to her place after that, and we talked about what was ahead for her. I very distinctly remember her saying that she was just playing house before, and now it was real. Very real. She now had to find a way to make ends meet and make sure the baby was taken care of. She was single and alone and forced into a world she wasn't ready for.

Around that time, I was also involved with the pregnancy of my friend that I'd known the longest. Her pregnancy was different because she was still in high school and living with her mom. Still trying to figure life out. Her boyfriend was one of those guys that everyone loves because he was a big goofball who was nice to everyone. He was a year older than us and had already graduated. He was the cliché guy you see in movies who hung out with guys who had already graduated but still hung around the high school and high school girls. He had no real plans for the future. All of his brothers were older than him, and they all seemed to have this same agenda. Just not much going for them in life. My friend didn't see this. She saw him as the perfect "fun" boyfriend. As a high school girl, there is nothing wrong with dating the carefree, no real future guy. In fact, he makes the perfect boyfriend. His mom always bought the beer and he somehow always had weed. What's not to love? However, as a pregnant teenager, these traits are the last things you want in a boyfriend. Unlike my former friend, these two didn't seem to have a plan. They didn't move out of their parent's house. They didn't move in together. They didn't plan. Just one day, they had a baby. Then, after the baby, their lives didn't really seem to change. We all still partied together and stayed up late. The baby would just come wherever with us. I'm sure there was a lot more to it than I knew or understood. That's just the thing, though. I didn't have to worry about it. I didn't have to understand.

Over time, I drifted from this group of friends and learned that eventually, the unseen stress of having the baby caught up with them. My friend is a smart girl and realized that maybe this guy wasn't the best baby daddy. He wasn't providing her the love and support she needed. Support the baby needed. She was lucky to have a family who acted as the support system when things fell apart with the not so great guy.

I'll take this time to say that those that get pregnant at a young age and decide to keep the baby are not judged by me. Every person lives their own life, faces the consequences of their actions and has to make decisions based on their life experience. The three friends that I mentioned here have all become amazing women. Even though it couldn't have been easy, they did it. They came out on top.

These experiences for me, as an outsider, were eye-opening. Between that and a few other friends having babies, I decided it was going to be a long time before I started a family. The idea that I would be stuck in a world that I was obviously not prepared for was not in my plan. But the pressure remained. It was still the expectation that I would get married and start a family. No one person put this pressure on me. It was just the way the world I grew up in was. I just decided to go onto my next step of leaving to college and seriously dating.

Chapter 5

College for me was... I don't even have a word for it. I initially had no intentions of going to college at all. I didn't know what I was "going to be when I grew up" and liked my job as a server. I had zero direction. Then, the majority of my friends up and left for college, and it hit me like a ton of bricks that I was not living a great life. I had been on my own for about six months and life was very hard, to say the least. Something needed to change. I had a jolt and decided to run off to college. I started classes a week late but I started. I also decided that I needed to get some friends and really dig into school; to start my life for real.

I attended Idaho State University in Pocatello, Idaho. I changed my major like three or four times and really didn't have a direction even though I craved one. I lived with my dad for a few weeks, and after that proved that would not work out, I moved in with my aunt and uncle who really took me under their wing. I started to get a focus. At the time attending church felt like a good way to find me some direction. I first started attending the "family ward" with my aunt and uncle and their three little girls. I had to dip my toe back into something that I hadn't done in a long time before really jumping in. I also started attending the Institute (church classes taught at the University) in hopes to just really grab onto anyone and to help guide me through this transition in my life. It was then that I decided to join the "Singles Ward".

The Singles Ward felt like a giant dating service with the goal of getting people married off. After I found the right ward, I made friends, and we had fun. Being single wasn't the end goal. Even though we were all single initially, the idea of marriage and family didn't go away. It's what we were taught and what we talked about. This teaching of "marriage is essential and raising a family is needed" in order to be complete just felt instinctual, so I didn't realize the effect it had on people. The effect it had on me.

Another factor that was focused on a lot was stay at home moms. I need to start by saying that there is nothing wrong with being a stay at home mom. It's a hard job that often seems impossible. It takes a strong woman to dedicate her whole life to her family and to make sacrifices to raise her children. If that is your career of choice, then I applaud you just as I would applaud a woman that decided to become a teacher or an astronaut or a doctor. That being said, I didn't really think about being one; I felt I was expected to be one. What would my community and family think of me if I didn't stay at home with my children?

Before I got married, I had thought seriously about becoming an OBGYN. I was in the room when one of my friend's babies was born, and it was, hands down, the most amazing experience of my life. Seeing life pop into the room was so overwhelmingly beautiful. I desired to be a part of that. I still wish I would have pursued this dream. As a freshman in college, I expressed to someone that I was thinking about pursuing this career. She instantly brought up how hard it was to have that job and have a family. How I would have to take a break in my career to raise my children and how maybe it wasn't the best job choice. Without realizing it, it slowly became obvious that the decision made for me was to be a stay at home mom. What is most alarming about this is I didn't even flinch at her comment. I had accepted that his career choice was mine. I never even thought about it. I even wrote a research paper in my English

102 class about my career choice of becoming a stay at home mom and why it was important.

Chapter 6

After a year of being in college, I decided that it was time to move out of my aunt and uncle's house. I found a flyer at the institute for a room for rent for $250. I met with the girl, decided it was a good fit and I moved in a week later. I became best friends with the "main" roommate and soon best friends with her two good friends. All we did was talk about boys and getting married. One friend had just come home from a Mormon mission and was on the warpath to find a guy to marry. One girl was waiting for a boy to come home from his Mormon mission so she could marry him. One friend was twenty-three, and since she didn't have a man in her life at all, was convinced that she was destined to be a spinster. It's not like we all disagreed about that. If you were not married by the time you were twenty-one and there was no boy on a mission you were waiting for, it seemed like a destiny of loneliness and lots of cats. I think it's natural for girls to focus on boys. Nothing wrong there. It is just another example of how much this idea that I should get married and start a family was prevalent in my life. And something I needed to do right away.

One thing to note about the town that I grew up in is the age this expected family was supposed to start. Most girls got married at the age of eighteen or nineteen, and boys got married at twenty-one. It didn't matter if they were still in school. They got married and made it work. My sister-in-law got engaged at the age of twenty-eight and married at twenty-nine. This is a healthy and normal age to get married. In my town, however, she was seen as at the end of her rope. Her pickings were slim. I asked her about this one time. She said that she was ok with not being married. She had no doubt great things were ahead for her. However, the world around her made her think she should feel otherwise. Older people in our community would look at her with concern and try to lift her spirits, saying all would be ok. She felt ok, but the community did not. When she got engaged, I announced it during a "good news minute" activity we had at church. I remember looking over at a friend of ours, and she sighed and mouthed, "Finally. Oh good." I remember feeling angry by that. Finally? The girl was twenty-eight! She was and is beautiful and fun and amazing to be around. She was going to find a husband, and if not, she would have been just fine. But we were in this world where it wasn't fine. She wasn't fine unless she was married and had a family. For some reason, when she finally did get to that point, it was like the world around us thought her life was just beginning and that for the last ten years she had been in limbo waiting. How unfair to her and the life she had lived up to that point. It was devalued because she had not met the expectations the world had set on her.

After a couple of years in college, I met a great guy, Michael. We were always kind of embarrassed when people would ask "How did you meet" because it was kind of lame. We met at church. Yes...that church where it was a dating service, we met there. At the time of meeting Michael, I was living with the previously mentioned girls in a house. In college you expect to live in a gross dorm or some run down house that students have live in for years. Not us, we were in an actually very nice house. Even though we didn't drink or smoke we were definitely the party house. We were always gathering everyone from church together to do some "crazy" stuff.

As a side note, the best memory in that house was the surprise birthday party for one of the roommates. We had so many people over. We played games, ate food, got in a huge cake fight (red frosting was stained into the floor and ceiling) and took a giant coed shower with our jeans on in the bathroom. Ah, what a good time.

Our parties didn't only include church members from our ward. My three best friends were into theater and did theater for the Institute. So, some of the friends that came over were also in this theater group. One of them being Sarah, a certain sister of a certain boy who had just come home from his Mormon mission. I got to know Sarah a little bit. I liked her.

One Sunday we were sitting in church and this boy gets up. Michael Hardy. He starts talking of his mission in Southern California and all he learned from it. At least I think. All I could focus on was how hot he was. I had seen him a couple of times at some church events. He would pull up in his blue car, blasting Blink 182, wearing a leather jacket. I always assumed the guy was way out of my league. And here he was. Standing up at the pulpit in a very nice suit and tie saying words I could not hear. I leaned over to my roommates and said, "Man this guy is hot!" They responded with, "That's Sarah's brother."

It. Was. Fate.

Somehow we created this grand plan of having a party one Monday night and inviting everyone. We would be sure to invite Sarah and lightly suggest that since her brother is newly home from his mission he should come to. It was a master plan. Everything backfired, as Michael was the only one that could come. Man it was super awkward. Like... so awkward. But we pushed through it.

Pretty instantly a friendship formed between us. Just friendship, because he was dating a girl who had been waiting for him to come home from that mission. Naturally, I was nothing but a lady and kindly waited on the side while he figured out what he wanted to do with this girl he wasn't totally into. For the record by "lady" I mean I texted him constantly and found every reason to hang out with him. He would help me study, go shopping with me, hang out, laugh; it was a good time. I will never forget the night he broke up with the girl he was dating. He called me and told me he was going to go and break up with her. The group of girls I was with decided that if he called me after the breakup, I was in. Guess what, he not only called, but came over. That's when I knew for sure that he liked me.

I wish I could say we instantly became boyfriend and girlfriend after this, but this is Michael we are talking about. I had to put in some more time. Soon after he broke up with his girlfriend, it was my birthday. We spent the whole night right next to each other. He even played with my hair. A couple of days later we held hands. Soon after that we kissed and, to spare the embarrassment of Michael, I will not tell you about our first kiss. I will just giggle to myself and always remember it fondly. It was soon after that we were standing in my doorway and I said, "If I were to introduce you to other people, how would I do that?" He said, "You can just say I'm Michael." He then left. I remember standing in the doorway for way too long being super upset. About 5 minutes later — which felt like an eternity — he said he realized he was an idiot and had to pull over on his way home. I got a text that read, "You can tell people I'm your boyfriend."

As all young, Mormon Idahoans do, soon after becoming boyfriend and girlfriend (I'm talking a couple months after), we started to talk about marriage. The real story of how it stopped being a hypothetical and became and actual, serious conversation, started on a Saturday. We were spending the day together and he started to ask me questions about finances and goals in life. That night, we were supposed to see Pirates of the Caribbean 2, but the line was so big we decided to bail and go to a park. It was there on the swings that we talked more seriously about it. Keep in mind marriage had come up quite a bit before. This was just a more in depth conversation. It was on those swings, in the dark, on a Saturday that we decided we were going to get married.

I remembered as he dropped me off I ran inside and no one was home. No. One. I had to sit on the couch and wait for someone to come home. Two of my roommates and two of our friends walked in and I jumped up and screamed, "I'm getting married!"

That week I went in and picked out the most gorgeous engagement ring. God I loved that ring. A few days after picking it out I got a call after a super bad day at work. Michael told me to meet him in the same park where we had talked the previous week. I got there and he was sitting on a table with his guitar. I sat down and he started to sing, "I'm sorry that it took so long to write this song, but I gave up. See one million words can't describe how it feels, to know your love…" I remember sitting there and thinking that this was it. I had to really decide whether or not I wanted to marry this very attractive, sweet, attentive man before me. A man who had declared his love to me so loudly I heard it throughout my whole body. A man who I loved with every piece of me. Who felt perfect for me. After his song he got down on one knee and said who knows what. Literally we both can't remember. What I do remember are the words, "Luanne Rose Evans, will you marry me?" I screamed yes at the top of my lungs. He slid the ring on my finger and I was shaking. We hugged and kissed. Some lady down at the other end of the park yelled "Congratulations." I was engaged. My life with my perfect partner was about to begin. The world that had been created for me of a stay at home mom with a lot of kids was ahead. I was going to start my family. We were married on December 1, 2006 in the Jordan River Temple in South Jordan, Utah. I was so happy that day. I remember at one point and time stopping and thinking about how happy I was to have married Michael. He had become my world and I was so excited to share that world with him.

Chapter 7

As I said, we got married on December 1st, 2006 in the Jordan River Temple in South Jordan, UT. There is a very clear memory I have while arm in arm with Michael walking down the sidewalk to a spot we were going to get pictures. I was in my wedding dress and as I walked I could feel the key to my locker that the temple workers had hooked on the inner layer of my dress way up by my thigh. I felt so happy. I could see my life was finally falling into place. I had found my family in Michael. He was going to support me and my children, we had decided on four, and life was good.

Even though we wanted them in the future, Michael and I decided before getting married that we were going to wait to have kids. I still didn't feel ready and remembered that reality was different with children. However, there seemed to be a different agenda in people's minds. A lot were surprised to find out I was on birth control. "When are the kids coming" was often a question I heard.

Soon after our wedding, we decided to trade in our cars to get a bigger, more reliable one. We wanted something that could drive in the snow well and something that wouldn't need to be fixed as often. We had a friend that was a cashier at the dealership, and while we were there, she asked us, with a wink, if we were preparing for anything. It was apparently time to have kids. The pressure was intense for me, and soon after getting married, I changed my mind and spent a month telling Michael I was ready to start a family. He gave in.

I can say with absolutely no doubt, Michael and I were not ready for kids. However, it seemed we just "had" to have them. It's only natural. Looking back now, I realize that it may be what's natural, but the insane pressure of having children for someone who can't have children is crushing. It makes me feel incomplete as a woman, and I have had to work really hard to accept that there is happiness without them. That there is a life after infertility. Even if you didn't grow up in a small Mormon town, it doesn't mean that you didn't experience the pressures and ideas of having a family. Perhaps you were expected to have a family and just like me that was that. So, when I am told that other people are happy without kids and I will probably be too, what is missing in that statement is the loss that comes with it. The expectation from the world and from your childhood and your whole understanding has to be worked through and let go before you can really be happy without kids. Even then, there will always be something missing.

It was soon after marriage when I began convincing Michael that it was time to have kids and that's where my infertility journey really started. It was from that moment that I started to understand the work and heartache of trying to have children.

My first six months of trying to get pregnant consisted of obsessively taking pregnancy tests and experiencing every single pregnancy symptom you could think of. Almost every month, I was late and convinced I was pregnant. To add to the disaster of those six months, I told everyone in the world that I was trying to have kids, and every month that I was convinced I was pregnant I'd tell them. Every month was met with disappointment and a new way to tell everyone I wasn't actually pregnant. In the meantime, my sister-in-law got pregnant. It was the first time I experienced that guilty twinge of being upset over someone's joy.

I also had a cousin that had a baby and a friend that found out she was pregnant. These became constant reminders that I wasn't. My implanted idea of starting a family was not coming to life and these new pregnancies were taunting reminders of just that.

As we grow older, we really start to understand the phrase "Keeping up with the Joneses." You can't help but compare your life to those around you just as my cousin did many years ago with her pregnant sister-in-law. I don't think it's always bad because it can drive you to become a better person, but clearly, it can get out of hand pretty fast. In the case of me and motherhood, I found myself comparing my childless life to others and thinking that maybe my life was out of sync.

It started to seem like everyone was pregnant. Everyone. Even the people you didn't think would be moms were pregnant and knitting baby blankets. Up until this point, our lives were on track together. We all went to college. We started getting married. We started moving away from our hometowns and beginning careers. But then it just took a turn. People were having babies left and right, and I was left baby-less. There was no way to keep up. I couldn't help but feel forgotten or like I wasn't meeting par.

During those first six months of trying, I was introduced to comments that people don't realize are rude. They believe they are just sharing their thoughts and ideas on the matter, but they don't realize and aren't sensitive to what is around them. I know I said these things to friends, and looking back, I feel bad. Because as the years go on, the comments cut deeper and feel harsher. The constant questions like "when are you going to have kids?" are just painful. It's like you want to scream "I AM TRYING!". These months were also when I started getting that advice I introduced in the beginning, like "just relax" and, "it will happen when you aren't worrying about it." Then there was one comment that a new mom said that still follows me wherever I go. As she was cradling her new baby, she told me that the family doesn't start until the baby is born. These are all words that seem encouraging and give you something to look forward to. However, these are words that actually cut deep. Very deep.

Looking back, I wish I noticed the signs. I mean, I was newly married so it's not like there was a lack of sex and I was doing the period math even with my 45 day and sometimes 60 day cycles. I wish I could see it wasn't normal to always be late or to have an unpredictable cycle. Maybe then I could have fixed it. Maybe then I could have stopped what was ahead. Young Luanne just didn't get it. Young is also a key word here. I was young. I did have time. We didn't think any biological clock was ticking. Plus, it HAD only been six months. No reason to see a doctor or really worry yet.

Eight months after getting married, Michael and I were presented with a new path. We had the opportunity to move to the Bay Area, and each go to schools that would help us get closer to our ideal jobs. For me this was culinary school and for Michael it was art school. In order to do this, we would have to go back to preventing pregnancy instead of the "not trying but not preventing" method. It was hard for me to accept, and I felt like I was betraying my family. By my family, I don't mean my sisters and mom and grandparents. I mean Michael and future children. I felt like putting my schooling first was wrong and selfish. I was excited about the road ahead, but I struggled. Even after we moved, I went back and forth with it a lot. We had discussed the stay at home mom thing by this point. Michael never pushed for it, but with the ideas implanted in my head - you are a woman, you are married, you must have kids, you must stay at home with them - I told him that it was what I wanted. It seemed like moving to California to go to culinary school would be counterproductive. My job was going to be a mom. Why was I betraying this decision by delaying what I thought I was supposed to do? Why was I so selfish?

Right before we moved, and I mean the week before we moved, I was the latest I had ever been. I was about two weeks late. Every single stick that I peed on was negative. However, the idea that I could be pregnant was there, and I needed to find out one way or another. If I was pregnant, everything we were planning for would have to be put on hold. Why would we move for me to go to school if I was pregnant and would then have to stay at home? I decided to go to a doctor, and get a blood test. Negative. Still no period, though.

A few days after the blood pregnancy test, Michael and I were at my in-law's house alone watching TV. I started to get a pain so sharp I couldn't even stand. I was crying and hurting, and Michael ran to the store to get pain killers. I sat at the kitchen table, doubled over with only one word coming into my mind: miscarriage. I was convinced. I knew the test had said negative, but at the time, I didn't really know if that was the most accurate way to find out if you were pregnant. I felt then like this was a miscarriage. Michael hugged me tight and told me it would be ok, but I couldn't know that. The pain soon subsided and a feeling of grief washed over me.

I decided it might be best to go to the doctor's office and took the next day off of work. Going in, the doctor didn't put me into a room with a gown as I had expected. Instead, she pulled me into her office. She spent about fifteen minutes telling me why I was stupid for thinking I was having a miscarriage. That the blood test had come back negative, and there was no way I was pregnant. That "The mere idea of a miscarriage was dumb." This is an exact quote from the doctor, by the way. She said instead, it was likely a cyst on my ovary that had burst. Again, young Luanne, why didn't you find out more about this? Why didn't you realize that this was an important and significant thing that needed to get checked? Maybe it was inevitable for me to be infertile. Maybe. Or maybe it wasn't, and these events could have been a wake-up call for me to get checked. Would the doctor have taken me seriously? Would they have helped me? I don't know. I'll never know because all I did was move forward knowing that I wasn't pregnant and that I was moving to a new city and starting the next chapter of my life.

Chapter 8

M oving to the Bay Area from a small town was absolutely unreal. We moved to a town that was in the process of going bankrupt, Vallejo, California. This is north in the Bay Area; about an hour or so from San Francisco. You cross two toll bridges to get to The City. Not only was Vallejo already going downhill, but we moved into the worst part of an already very dangerous town. When people I worked with found out where I lived, it was always followed by wide eyes and a list of things to do if attacked. I'm not exaggerating.

My in-laws helped us move, and the first day, we unpacked and ate pizza. The next three days were filled with an insane amount of anxiety and hell. To fully explain, I first need to let you dive a little more into the mind of a crazy person, a.k.a. me. You pick up a million things from your parents. Some are genetic, like their nose or toes or body shape. Other things are learned behaviors, like when and how to talk about poop or what's considered funny. I picked up a lot and can confidently say I am an equal mashup of both Mom and Dad. One thing I picked up (and grew) was the inability to go with the flow. I am a planner.

I fully and totally believe that everything should have a specific plan, and if not completed correctly, the world just simply stops turning. It took me years and years to realize that this caused insane stress and anxiety attacks that resulted in me yelling and throwing things. At the peak of my anxiety attacks, I stopped talking altogether. I am not a professional about this stuff but I think I don't talk because I can't handle the chaos. My body and mind simply shut down because it's too much for me to handle. Over the years, I have gotten better at recognizing, understanding and reacting to these anxiety attacks. But at that point in my life, moving from a small town to the Bay Area, I had no understanding that it was anxiety at all. However, it was with that move that my world turned to chaos.

We arrived in Vallejo on a Friday, I was scheduled to start school the following Monday after moving in. I had to go into The City to learn my route to get to school via public transportation and go to orientation. I started my day by discovering that I had to first go to the docks and pay $450/month for a public transportation pass. That pass got me on an hour boat ride from Vallejo to Pier 1 in San Francisco. From there, I had to run two blocks to catch a bus at the right number. From that bus, I would get off at my stop and run down three blocks to arrive at one campus. Then, a school shuttle would take me from the campus in the Tenderloins to the campus in Presidio. It took us four small-towners about six hours to figure this out. We walked all over the city and asked a million people a million questions. I was 100% sure I would have no idea what to do on Monday.

Through some sort of strange luck, we made it to my orientation. I got excited for the next two years ahead and felt like even though I didn't really know how to get to school, I would enjoy it once I got there. On our way back, we ran into some pretty bad traffic, and after getting off the school shuttle, we went in search of a city bus. Before I go on, let me make sure this picture is painted correctly.

I grew up in a small town.

With almost no diversity.

90% of the people living there shared the same Christian religion and went to church on Sunday.

The worst drug I personally knew anyone had done was weed. I believed the videos that told me that only scary people do any drugs "harder" than that.

Swearing by adults was almost never heard in public. Sometimes you might hear a slip now and again.

I grew up in a bubble. What's worse is, it was a bubble I didn't even know existed. In high school, I was pretty "rebellious," and by rebellious, I mean, I smoked cigarettes, drank alcohol, smoked some weed, cut classes and swore. I legitimately thought I was the ultimate badass and was breaking all the rules. That's right. All. The. Rules.

Picture painted?

So, four people from a small town are out in the city looking for the bus during what turned out to be San Francisco's Love Day parade. This was nothing like I had ever seen in my life. Everyone was under the influence of something. The smell of weed and alcohol smothered the street. And there were people dancing everywhere. I remember wanting to only look at the ground but having to look up every once in a while. When I did, the sites were horrendous to my sad, sheltered eyes. There were naked women dancing in cages. There were fat, naked men walking around and letting it all hang out. There were images that, to this day, even though I am far from that little sheltered girl walking the streets of a Love Day parade, are scarred in my memory and cannot be shared.

With our heads down, the four of us managed to make it back to the ferry to get us back to our small, dangerous apartment in a town where we knew no one.

I was dead silent the whole way home. I remember my father-in-law asking me questions. I knew he knew I was worried. I tried to answer the shortest way I could, but I was having one of my worst anxiety attacks to date. What the hell had I done? I moved thousands of miles away. I stopped the growth of the number of people in my family. I had uprooted everything I knew and everything that felt familiar to what felt like the city of Sodom and Gomorrah. Just to wander around, trying to find where to go to school and still not even know. I felt we had made the right decision when moving. It was exciting to spread our wings, but man was I scared. Nothing was going according to plan, and I didn't know how it was going to work out. I was so anxious the next few days. I'm sure I was on edge and very snappy to Michael. It was overwhelming to feel like we were going up against something so unknown and unfamiliar.

However, we did it. We survived. I did make it to school on time that Monday. I even made friends with the bus driver who would take me through the homeless ridden parts of the City and make me feel safe. I sincerely enjoyed school. My experiences were so different and I really started to see a new world.

There are about a million and one things in the Bay Area that are different from living in my small town. I had to get used to a lot. People being openly gay and swearing on the street, wearing "skimpy" clothes and the sheer number of bars felt very different. I think it would be the same if someone went the opposite direction, from a big city to a small town. They would be shocked by the slow pace and the general conversations that can revolve around one giant store, Wal-Mart. Culture shock is a real thing, and it takes time to adjust to all the differences.

I could make a longer list of the differences between small towns and big cities. But one of the biggest differences was the questions we were asked as a couple. Instead of "so when are you having kids," we started hearing "YOU ARE ALREADY MARRIED? But you are so young!" Guys, I got married at nineteen. It was normal and accepted and, as I mentioned earlier, expected for me to get married at this age. To go from that to people not even comprehending the idea that I was married was really hard and frustrating. People often asked if it was because I found out I was pregnant or if it was because Michael was in the military. I would then have to take time to explain that where I came from, the idea of me being too young to get married was unheard of. That I was the normal age. After a certain amount of time, I just started saying, "Yup. Young." It was easier to let it go.

Naturally, since people were already appalled that I was married, they were definitely not asking about kids. It was a relief. Suddenly, my life didn't have to focus on becoming a mom and all of the unanswered questions that came with it. I could focus on school, Michael's school and our marriage.

We lived in Vallejo for only about six months. Then we moved to a small town called Emeryville. This town is on the other side of the Bay Bridge from San Francisco. Over time, we realized we were not in any type of evil city. Just a city that was different than the small town I grew up in. Michael started at a private art school. We made friends and somehow made it work. In fact, even though I have zero intentions of ever living there ever again, the Bay Area still feels like home a little. A lot of my friends live there. And I can safely say I know Oakland and The City pretty well and can get around without Google Maps to reach most places. The Bay Area has a part of me.

During this time, friends from high school were all getting married and having kids. And I slowly started to realize how different our lives were becoming from those at home. Our goals and outlooks started to drift in different directions. So many people from high school were buying homes and becoming parents. Women were dropping out of school and staying at home with their children. Instead, I was worried about grades. Graduating. Finding an interrnship and knowing whether or not I was going to be a baker or a chef. Becoming a parent was so far off in the distance, I had stopped thinking about it all together...

Until suddenly, something shifted, and everything seemed closer.

Chapter 9

After graduation, I was working as a baker. Michael was close to graduating, and it felt like becoming real grown-ups was getting closer. With that shift, I started to think about children again. I started to turn back into that small-town girl. I was ready for my white picket fence, working husband and babies while I stayed at home and cooked and cleaned. At the same time, I was excited for ideas ahead in my career. I saw the worth in what I was doing and started to see the impact. Plus, I was damn good at it. I was one of the best. I saw clear stepping stones into my future as a career person. I also had ideas for some businesses that I felt would be successful. But every time I combated these opposing ideas in my mind, I would call myself crazy. Of course, being a stay at home mom was all I wanted. I was taught this growing up. I saw the benefits of having my mom home with us. I noticed a difference in the times she worked. I mean, it's what you did, right? It's what all of my sisters-in-law did. It's what my friends did. Was I wrong for thinking any other way?

So, Michael was close to graduating from school. And around that time was when we stopped preventing pregnancy again. I don't remember what pushed us over the edge. He was reluctant. He was worried about money and getting a job. Where were we going to live? How would we live on one salary? I wasn't reluctant. I mean, I had started the conversation! But I was nervous. Living in the Bay Area was and is insanely expensive. Everyone I knew had a dual income, and most were either really successful lawyers or lived in a small apartment. How would we make this work? I wasn't sure but the time had come. We had decided we would hold off until we graduated and now, we were there. The natural timeline led us to this moment of accepting. We were going to be parents.

A few years before, something happened to me that is worth noting. I almost died. Not like, "Haha, I totally almost died." Like, "It's amazing I am living" almost died. We moved from Vallejo to Emeryville during my Spring Break in April. After we moved in, I got very ill. I assumed it was because I was working two jobs and going to school. I figured my body was catching up with me. Right after what felt like the flu left, I started to get some very weird symptoms. First came thirst. I was always thirsty. Like overwhelmingly could never get enough water thirsty. Naturally, with drinking a lot of water, my urination increased. Plus, over time, my urine started to smell sickly sweet. In the middle of the night, I would wake up with insane charley horses. My symptoms started to get worse. In the beginning of August I had a really bad yeast infection. With lack of insurance and a need to combat the infection I went to Planned Parenthood. I weighed 135 pounds when they weighed me. They got me some medication and told me to come back in three weeks to follow up. Three weeks later, I went in, they weighed me again, and I was 115 pounds. In three weeks, I lost twenty pounds. Around this same time my hair started falling out excessively. I remember comparing the amount of hair I had lost by brushing it to my wedding ring. The amount of hair was about the size of my fist and I wore a size 4 ring. Last symptom, I was hot. One of the last nights at home, before going to the hospital, I slept with ice cubes.

I remember the day I finally went to the hospital well. That morning, I woke up and was so hot and thirsty and tired. I couldn't take it anymore, so I went to Baskin Robins and got an ice cream cone. I sat in the car with the AC on full blast and ate the ice cream. It didn't help. I drove to work, which was, at the time, a restaurant where everyone hated me (yes everyone) and sat in the parking lot. I remember calling my mom and asking her to look up symptoms to help me figure out what was going on. She told me to go to the hospital. But I got out of my car and went into work. My supervisor asked how I was doing. I told her I wanted to go to the hospital then walked away and clocked in. After about an hour, she sat me down and asked me what was going on. I told her all of the symptoms I had been having. I almost passed out talking to her. She was definitely annoyed with me and my symptoms but told me to go to the hospital. So, I picked up Michael and went.

The hospital was busy when we arrived. Yet despite that, after triage, I was only in the waiting room for fifteen minutes before they called me back. By now, I weighed ninety pounds, a frail look for my 5'4" frame. I slipped into the gown and waited for the nurse who had trouble getting a blood sample. Next, I waited for the doctor who came in and said, "You have diabetes. It's something you will have to deal with for the rest of your life." Then walked out. I had untreated diabetes for so long that I ended up in a state called Diabetic Ketoacidosis (or DKA). They say the perfect blood sugar is 124. My blood sugar at this point? Over 981. My blood was so thick that they had a hell of a time getting it out of me and had to every four hours. It is a miracle I wasn't in a coma because if I had fallen into a coma, I would have died.

I spent five days in the ICU. I had to learn how to inject needles into myself, and people kept coming and giving me classes. By the time I went home, I felt better than I had in a long time. It took quite a few months with a good friend who has Type 1 as well (she was a better teacher than anyone else - you know who you are and you are amazing!), but I learned how to manage it. I'm not perfect now, but I do amaze new doctors with the knowledge of my disease and the ways I treat it. The truth is, I will most likely die from diabetes one day. I will get old, and it will get harder to manage, and one day, it will get the best of me. Before that happens, I want to be as healthy as I can be. So, I am always sure to know what is going on with my body.

I want to note this because what had happened to my body was very damaging in a lot of different ways. Every part of my body was affected and not everything bounced back. Type 1 Diabetes (which is different than Type 2, and thus has nothing to do with my weight or bad eating habits) is an auto-immune disease. Your body starts attacking itself, so mine killed my pancreas, which also affects my kidneys and liver. It's safe to believe that other things were destroyed in the process.

Now, back to the story. I had decided to stop preventing.

The timeline gets a little fuzzy for me here. I don't remember becoming crazy obsessive with the pregnancy tests at first, but that just simply doesn't sound like me. I remember being late a lot (I mean, c'mon it's me), and I remember hoping for symptoms. I think, though, the first few months I was just coasting. Hopeful, but not devastated. Also, we were so poor that buying pregnancy tests every month was just not in the budget. I do remember that after a few months, I started getting antsy. I was smarter this time around about a few things. First, not everyone in the world knew I wanted to get pregnant. Next, as mentioned with the tight budget thing, I didn't buy as many pregnancy tests. Also, I did more period math and made sure we were doing the baby dance on the right days.

A lot was happening, but I do remember a few things. One of those things was having a conversation in a car with one of my friends, Brandy. It was the first time I had really talked about kids with a Bay Area friend. Everyone there was so unfocused on it that it just never came up. However, Brandy and I were in the same spot in our lives, so I think it came up naturally. She told me that the way they were preventing was by not practicing "safe sex." She said she was worried that she actually couldn't get pregnant. I told her there was more to it than sex, that destiny and fate had a lot to do with it.

We'll take a brief time out in a moment to talk about my belief in fate. You will learn that it's a big part of this story. I shared with her that we were not preventing, but not for how long (at this point, it was longer than I was comfortable with). She just wished me the best, and we didn't discuss it again for a long time, which I'll also talk about later.

Another thing I remember was a new couple that moved into our area and started going to church with us. She was speaking in a Sunday meeting and shared with us that she and her husband were unable to have kids. She shared that she didn't really know what the future held for her, but she was pretty sure it would not hold children. I felt devastated for her. I didn't know anyone who couldn't have kids. I just had that small memory of my cousin, as mentioned before, and that was it.

Soon after that, it seemed infertility became more prevalent. Part of it was that this friend was so brave to tell her story to the whole congregation that it opened the door for more women there to talk about not being able to have children. In addition to that, one of my roommates from college disclosed to me that she was having a lot of health problems, and it seemed she could not have kids. I very vividly remember telling her all the wrong things. "Well, you can just adopt, right?" and, "Oh, I'm sure it will happen." Even "You know if you stop thinking about it, it will happen in no time." Remember, those are bad friend things to say to someone who tells you that they can't have kids. Don't ever say them.

Overall, this idea of pregnancy, more importantly, not getting pregnant, became more and more around me. It started glaring at me, reminding me that I was not getting pregnant to the point where I was starting to get sad and worried.

One day my sister-in-law called. She told me about some struggles she had getting pregnant and then told me, "I'm sorry, I'm pregnant." I cried. She cried. We cried together. Besides the first time finding out my other sister-in-law was pregnant, back when Michael and I were first married, this is the first time I really felt sad about another pregnancy. It's the first time it really set in that I was not pregnant. For reasons unknown, it was challenging to get pregnant. Yet, other people could get pregnant. People who already had kids. People who already knew the joy of motherhood. I was sad and angry. But I was in denial of these feelings. How horrible of a person do you have to be to be mad at someone who is pregnant? This sister was the beginning of a very long list of people I am close to who got pregnant. Each announcement, even of strangers, became more of a stab to the heart. This one was just the beginning of the darkness and loneliness that surrounded pregnancy announcements. Like I said, though, I shrugged it off. When the sisters would call with more pregnancy announcements, they always started by saying they were sorry. I hated that. Why should people have to be sorry? Why did their sorry not make me feel any better? What was wrong with me? Those are all things I thought of often.

As time passed, I just kept thinking about fate. Oh, fate. My whole life, I have believed that things happen for a reason. That every trip and stumble in this road we call life was for a reason. My friend from high school once told me that she didn't believe in fate. She didn't like the idea of her life being decided for her. I thought she was crazy. I kept telling myself that it just wasn't my time to have kids yet. That things were going to have to happen in order for me to get pregnant. Every month came with an excuse as to why it wasn't that month. I was just waiting and waiting for fate.

As I shared my struggles with a few more friends, not many, they would tell me the same thing. "Oh, it's just not the right timing yet." I even came up with this idea that I was grateful. Grateful that I wasn't like all those girls I knew in high school that got pregnant when it wasn't the right time. I was lucky because God was waiting until the timing was absolutely perfect for me.

I have been talking a lot about the past, but just for a moment, I'm going to bring you into the present day.

I am now to a point where I simply don't know what to think about this idea of fate. These days, it's hard for me to believe that things had to happen or have to happen for me to get pregnant. I know I believe a series of events have taught me a lot, and I have learned a lot about myself. I know I believe that if it wasn't for certain events, like infertility, I wouldn't be at the place I am now. However, I also know that if I didn't have infertility, I would have learned different lessons that would have been equally important, and I would be in a place that would be "perfect" for my situation. The lessons would have been relevant to whatever situation I was in. It just happens that because I'm infertile, I learn the lessons that come with being infertile. Just like someone who has kids. They learn lessons about being a parent. Whatever situation you are in forces you into the lessons that come with it.

The idea of fate and my lack of understanding or faith in it makes me sad. Fate, to me, is linked to the idea of a higher power; in my case, a Heavenly Father. From what I was taught, fate is because our Father in Heaven knows everything and sees everything. He affects different parts of our lives to guide us to be better people. So, my lack of ability to have faith in fate these days connects to the lack of my ability to have faith in a Heavenly Father. I still do believe in a Heavenly Father – I think -, but at times, I think he has forgotten me, and the "fate" I am supposed to have. This has led to a lack of ability to think that anyone up there cares for me or is guiding my life for the better. Losing the idea of fate is one heart-wrenching and horrible side effect of infertility. I miss believing that I'm holding out for something great. I miss the idea of, "oh, this is the path that is perfect for me." I'm on no path. I'm just a human living life and because of circumstances, I'm forced to face other circumstances. Trust me when I say there is nothing perfect about what is here for me.

Sometimes when I sit and think about infertility, I feel like I'm looking into a black hole in my heart. Like I'm seeing positive feelings of the past sucked into an area I not only can't get to, but don't really want to. Losing faith in fate is one of those things. I stare at it, and can't even remember the joy of holding out for this great path in front of me. How did I ever have this joy? How is it possible to have happiness about something that is so sorrowful? It's a feeling that is easy to lose, though. No matter who you are. If you want kids. Don't want kids. Are married. Are single. If you are a woman, you expect that the moment you decide to have kids, you will have kids. Not for one minute do you stop to think otherwise. Especially when that's piled onto a past and the idea that your calling in life is to become a mother. That you will be a mom. Your community, your church and your family expects it. How can I have faith in this idea that there is something like fate out here to help me?

In the movie Forrest Gump, he talks about this exact thing. He says that his momma always taught him to believe in fate and "destiny." That life was laid out before him, and he just needed to take what was there. He said he always felt his life was like a feather, just floating through the air and landing where it will. However, at the end of the movie he says that now he thinks it may be both. That both the idea that there is a path for you and that you kind of float around to get there are truths. I think that's where I'm at now- no longer at "perfect" faith that someone or something is guiding me to exactly where I need to go, and at the end is a baby. I do think I am led to certain areas in work and life, to find solutions to problems and struggles, but I no longer think my end is a baby.

However, looking back, fate was all I had to keep me moving forward.

Chapter 10

I remember after a few months I was starting to get nervous, and I felt a little scared. But, I hadn't given much thought to being infertile. My mom always joked how she was a "fertile myrtle" who could get pregnant if my dad simply looked at her. I assumed this meant infertility wouldn't be something I would have to worry about.

On my fifth-year wedding anniversary, I remember thinking a lot about parenting. Five years is a big milestone, so we decided to do more than just the dinner to celebrate. We did go out to dinner but then also went to an arcade and rode go-karts. It was so fun. As we were leaving the arcade, I told Michael that this anniversary would probably be the last one without kids, so I was happy we did what we did. I was so sure it was just around the corner.

My timeline stops becoming fuzzy at a key point. Our friends, who we shall call Sally and Jack, moved into the area and started attending church with us. Sally was newly pregnant, and Jack was finishing med school. We hit it off with these two right away. They lived pretty close by, and we hung out with them often. They were always a hoot. I don't remember exactly how or when we found out, but they shared that Sally had become pregnant through fertility treatment. She was very open about it and talked about it often. I don't know if she talked about it often to everyone, but she sure did to me. We were close, so it made sense that she would share intimate details with me. She explained the process of infertility. The trying. The failures each month. The sadness. The acceptance. Then the first step. She got pregnant through a process called IUI. My doctor explained it to me the best way. You put the egg in a very large building with lots of rooms. Instead of the sperm wandering the streets of the town looking for the egg, you show the sperm the building the egg is in and shove it in the front door. The sperm is still required to look for the egg and guess the right room, but at least it's in the door. Sally told me all the steps that were required to get this process done, and she was the first friend I opened up to about how I wasn't getting pregnant. In fact, she was the first person I really opened up to about fears. I think I was admitting them really out loud to even myself. She listened. She understood.

Sally has been a good and important friend to me for a lot of different reasons. However, she will never know nor understand the importance of her friendship to me, specifically when it comes to infertility. By telling me all of her struggles, and her processes, she helped me feel brave. Infertility is lonely. Taking that first step and accepting that something might be wrong is hard and terrifying. You just don't know what is on the other side of that door, and you don't want to know. Sally helped me through it though. Without her even realizing it, I saw options on the other side because of her. I saw the process, and I could process it. I talked to her more about her infertility than she probably wanted to. She would often reassure me that everything would likely be fine, and I would probably be pregnant in six months. I know she believed that. It actually was that belief, and the fact that it wasn't happening, that pushed me over the edge to consider opening up to someone in the medical field about it.

I try really hard to be a Sally to others these days. Hell, I'm writing this book to do just that. I have had quite a few friends reach out to me and share their struggles. We cry together. We share frustrations together. Most of them are "closet" infertility sufferers that need an outlet. I believe I am that outlet. I have two very close friends, and we talk all day, every day through messenger. At one point in time, they both were actively trying to get pregnant unsuccessfully. Each month, I could feel their frustration more. One friend said, "I have been doing this for just a couple of months, and I am freaking out. I don't know how you do it, Lu." Both of them eventually got pregnant, but it was nice to know I was there until then. I was prepared to help them through this door and to the other side to begin a rough journey. I think it's important when you are struggling with something as real and as hard as infertility to find a Sally who knows the scariness of it.

Without Sally realizing it, she is the reason I talked to my doctor about my infertility. Unfortunately, he was no help at all. He taught me about period math and sent me on my way. It wasn't enough for me; I had been doing period math for months. In addition, my periods had started to be even more unpredictable. At one point, my cycle was thirty days, then sixty days, then ninety. It even got up to one hundred and twenty days one cycle.

I found a fertility clinic that didn't require referrals and decided to schedule an appointment. Crossing over the line from suspecting something might be wrong to accepting there might be something wrong is hard. Even if it has taken months or years, and you are not pregnant, you rationalize it. You may be worried and scared, and in the back of your mind, you know you need to see a doctor, but you push forward with this idea that everything is ok. It takes a strong woman to decide there might be something wrong. And it is terrifying to admit. If there might be something wrong, it means you might get news that you can never have kids. If you seek fertility treatment, you have to accept that there is a chance you might hear the worst. It's just the truth, and why so many women suffer for years without help. I went about seven or eight months before I accepted it. Even then, as I was driving to my first appointment, I had to breathe through it. I sat in the parking lot for a few minutes, trying to gain the courage to go in. Sitting in the waiting room, I thought about bolting. The pressure of it all was too much. The want to have a child won, though, and I stayed.

Since starting my journey with infertility, I have had six different infertility doctors. Each doctor has been better than the previous one. This first doctor was not only the worst of the six but just the worst in general. She did very little testing on me, shared no results, did not test Michael and immediately set me up for IUI. She did not explain what IUI was, by the way. She just assumed since I was young, I could get pregnant and that I was a little impatient about the whole thing. I had even told her that my cycles were thirty, sixty and then ninety days, but she didn't think anything of it. She just told me we would proceed with a procedure when I was ready.

A few days after this appointment, my friend, Brandy, the one I had first discussed this with, randomly called me. She said that it sounded crazy, but she had something for me. It turned out that her insurance had some type of something (I mean honestly who really gets anything about insurance) and they had to spend a certain amount of money by the end of the year. She had remembered our conversation and felt that maybe she should buy us an ovulation tracker. Not a cheap one, but one of those super high-tech fancy ones. She told me I couldn't say no, and it was already heading to my house. Amazing, right? Yeah, she's amazing. We decided to give it a try. In three months, I ovulated one day. Something was wrong. I couldn't deny it anymore.

We decided that going through the procedure with the bad doctor was the way to go.

Between originally going to the doctor, using the ovulation tester and deciding to go through with the procedure, a new adventure was starting to head our way. And like everything, it has a backstory.

When I was a girl, I lived in San Diego for about three years. I remember the smell of hot rain on the pavement, the warm winter months, a non-stop summer feel, going to the zoo and SeaWorld often and fun beach trips. I loved San Diego. My dad's family lived there and my neighbor, who was my best friend. When Michael was in high school, he traveled to San Diego during a choir tour and fell in love with the city. His need to be near the ocean and to fulfill that inner surfer that always called to him was met there, and it was definitely on our radar as a destination for living. We longed for it.

Right around the time we had decided to go forward with the procedure, Michael got a phone call. His previous boss had moved down to San Diego just a few months earlier and set up a department at the University of San Diego. He needed someone with Michael's skill set, and after a trip there and an interview, he offered Michael a job. Even though this sounds like a shoe-in for us getting to live somewhere we always wanted to, it wasn't that easy of a decision. We had a life in the Bay Area. We both had good jobs, great benefits, amazing friends. I knew how to get to the grocery store and the church and anywhere really. It was our home. Even though we didn't love living there because of the crime, the cost of living, and the overall vibe that was a little too much for us, I didn't want to leave something comfortable behind. We really had to weigh out our pros and cons. One day, though, we decided we better move forward with it. It was a good opportunity, and the timing felt right. We decided we would leave the Bay Area on December 29th.

After deciding our leave by date, I contacted the bad doctor's office and let them know of our plans. I asked if they would still be able to do the procedure despite Christmas and the now small timeline before we moved. They said I would be able to do the procedure but would have to immediately follow up with a doctor in San Diego. It all felt right. Like my life was falling into place. We were moving to the city where I never thought we could actually live and soon I would be pregnant. All the "signs" pointed to this being a part of that plan I assumed was in place for me.

To start my procedure, the first thing I had to do was take a pill for ten days. It was a progesterone pill (I later learned, since my doctor didn't share any information with me at the time), and after the ten days, I started my period. Soon after my last day, I went in for an ultrasound. They found a cyst on my ovary and told me the procedure would have to wait until the ovary cyst went away. Meaning, it wasn't going to happen this cycle.

One of the things I hate most about infertility doctors is how callous they can be. They are surrounded by infertility, so they become numb to it. It seems as if they don't realize we are sitting in their offices, spending every penny we have, holding onto hope and a prayer. This doctor was especially insensitive. Again, I am pretty sure she just thought I was an impatient young lady who was going to get pregnant instantly. She didn't realize that I wasn't. She didn't realize that the way she told me it wasn't going to happen that month would affect me deeply; that I would cry my whole way home, not knowing who else to cry to. She didn't realize that, in secret, I would be so sad that what seemed like the right path I thought I was on was instead a bump in the road. A bump leading to false hope and crushed dreams.

I know what a lot of you may be thinking. You could have cried to your husband. Or to your mom and your friends. Unfortunately, it's not that easy. There is nothing that anyone can ever say in this life to help you with the pain of finding out an infertility treatment didn't work. Why would I burden someone with the upset and sad feelings I have if they can't comfort me? I couldn't even express what I wanted to say. It's impossible to speak the words of your heart. You are feeling incomplete, unworthy to be a woman, scared of the future and like a failure all wrapped up in one. You feel an insane amount of anger, but you have no idea who to be angry at. All you can do is cry. Talking to Michael didn't feel easy. In fact, it feels ten times worse to share it with him because you are afraid of what he may be thinking. Will he decide that maybe it's better to be with someone who can have kids? Will he think I'm silly for being so sad?

Being told a treatment didn't work traps you in your emotions, with no instruction manual on how to get out. You just have to learn to breathe and cry through it, hoping that the "magical" path is ahead of you and that fate has something else in store for you.

For this first failed fertility treatment, I managed to cry, take a deep breath and recover. With the move to San Diego very close in the future, I was able to bury my thoughts and feelings under the items going into moving boxes. I was convinced that San Diego was where everything would fall into place, and it all was going to be ok. Little did I realize how wrong I was.

Chapter 11

A little less than a year before moving to San Diego, we decided it was that time. We thought about it. We talked about it. We considered our options. We realized it was just time. So, we got a dog.

Roxy is a German Shepherd/ Catahoula Leopard Dog crazy bouncing bean. If you don't know much about either of those breeds just know they are both high energy and too smart for their own good dogs. Roxy is crazy. As a puppy I don't think she ever slept. Michael would wake up with her in the early morning hours to take her outside. He would then come back in and lay on the floor to take a short nap before getting up for the day. During this time Roxy would grab both strings of his hoodie and pull them as tight as they would go so all you could see was Michael's nose sticking out and she would tug and tug and tug on those the whole time Michael slept. Without realizing it, Roxy was something in my life that was filling a void. This void first started with my first failed fertility treatment and it would grow as time went on. Roxy's bouncy and "mind-of-their-own" ears along with her sweet personality and amazing sleeping positions would provide me with love of a child that I was missing in my life.

The actual move to San Diego was funny. We had found a place to live but really had no idea what we were moving into. We saw some pictures and looked on Google Earth, but it was a total unknown. We had heard that there is no "bad part of town" in San Diego, so we were just winging it. When driving from the Bay Area as we got closer and closer to our new place, San Diego just got prettier and prettier. As it turns out, we were moving to one of the nicer areas. The place wasn't amazing, big or anything we would want to live in forever. But, the area was nice, and I was about a two-minute drive to work and other great spots. We had signed up for a six-month lease, and during that time, it definitely worked.

Once we got to San Diego, we both had about two weeks before our jobs started. We spent those days at the zoo, the beach, on hikes, downtown, et cetera. We really got to enjoy San Diego, and it was fun. Our first night there was New Year's Eve. We had zero belongings (because they were coming on a moving truck) and nowhere to go. So, we blew up our air mattress and watched Tom Hanks movies until midnight. Those first ten days were nice, and when our stuff arrived, we were able to unpack and settle in before starting work.

Moving to San Diego was all about Michael and the job he had. In the Bay Area, I had worked my way up to Assistant Manager at a bakery-cafe chain, and luckily, the franchise in San Diego had a spot for me. They welcomed me with open arms. I transitioned with the same company to different areas twice in my life, and there is no good way to say it; it sucks. I can't pinpoint exactly what it is, but there is just something about trying to find your value in a new place that is hard. It seems like you have to find a way to prove yourself right away. But, you barely even know where the bathroom is, so doing that is challenging. You also tend to get lost. Not like wandering around work, but like lost in the shuffle. Your new boss recognizes that you can do your job, and doesn't feel a need to baby you through it, but you need that daily connection, so you feel remembered. Another challenge is the feeling that you have no allies. No one to go to so you can complain. No one to ask the more "embarrassing" questions on the stuff you should know but just don't. As a manager, you have no employee you can turn to when the shift is going down, and you need help bringing it up. As a new manager, employees tend to be standoffish. They know nothing about you, and they have their "thing" going so they don't want it interrupted. They don't know yet if you are nice or mean or lenient or strict. And the whole thing ends up feeling lonely.

This move was the first time I moved within a company, and it took me a long time to figure it out. I had reached out to the general manager a couple of times, and she was nice and did what she could, but the problem was that I didn't know what I needed. Looking back at both of my transitions within a company, I wonder if there is anything anyone can do. I think you just have to go through the loneliness.

Eventually, I made it through. I had to let time pass, and my outgoing personality break through the barriers of unsure employees. It's funny to look back now because I became so integrated in that restaurant, I can't believe I ever felt like I didn't belong.

Settling into San Diego for me, once past the first rough patch, was fairly easy. I worked alongside a few women with the youth at church, and they were really friendly and welcoming. We would go on morning walks and talk during church. We would share love and thoughts with each other. It was nice. Mira Mesa, where we lived, was a great area. It was fairly small, so it was easy to learn how to get around. Slowly, it felt more and more like home.

For Michael settling in seemed to settle in fairly well and quickly. The team he worked with was small and they were, essentially, creating the online department so it seemed work was fun for him. He is an introvert so putting him in this environment for work was a good way for him to make friends. He really enjoyed the commute because of the scenery, and we were constantly trying to find different things to do during the weekend because we felt like our options were endless. We felt like we were home.

San Diego may have felt like home, but the apartment we lived in really didn't. It was Roxy's first apartment, and she struggled with the noise from neighbors. We were on the top floor, but people walking by and our neighbors were often heard. Living on the top floor had very little benefits. We didn't have to hear the stomps of upstairs neighbors, but it was hot, and we had to take Roxy out at least two times a day. Carrying up groceries was also pretty horrible. I was constantly counting down the days until we could move again.

It was great to have Roxy in my life. However, it was becoming time to reassess and move forward. After we got settled in and figured out our benefits, it became time to start thinking about my infertility again and what we were going to do. I went to see a doctor, expecting to pick up where I had left off. I told him everything my previous doctor had said, which was pretty much nothing and asked him to do whatever treatment I was planning on doing. With that, hopefully, boom! A baby on the way! Of course, nothing is ever that easy.

This second doctor of my treatment was very different from my first. He explained everything to me and in ways that made sense. He really did seem to care and wanted me to really know and learn what it was that was happening and why.

The first thing I learned was that there are many ranges of infertility. Male and female infertility. In those two columns are what feels like countless possibilities of what could be going on. It ranges from the "easier" stuff, like an irregular cycle or low sperm count, to things like a thin uterine lining or lack of eggs. Sometimes it's like everything rolled into one. With this information came steps of what we needed to do.

First, we needed to identify the problem. To discover this, we had to get blood work done, get a couple of ultrasounds (some more painful than others) and check Michael's sperm. It was a lot of testing.

Testing is probably one of the most asked questions I get. "What do they test?" "How quickly will I know?" "Do tests define the problem 100%?" Again, this is my journey and my journey alone. So these are the tests I had. Other tests may exist that I don't know about and science has surely progressed so there may be something else there. These are the tests I took and what they discovered for my journey. Everyone else's will be parallel in some ways and completely different in another. The following tests are my story.

We were lucky. I cannot emphasize enough how lucky we were. All of our tests were covered by insurance. The testing alone would have been thousands and thousands and thousands of dollars if it wasn't for our insurance. Some couples can't even get past this first hump because they don't have the money. Money is a very real part of infertility. It's the unspoken grim reaper of hope in an already trying time period.

So, what were they testing for? Even though this doctor was not the best, most amazing doctor I had, he is at the top of my list. I am a person who needs to hear frank and realistic information. He was very thorough and didn't sugar coat anything. He answered any questions I had and walked me through every step of the way. Which means, he was able to tell me exactly what they were testing me for.

First, they had to find out why I wasn't having regular cycles. In order to do this, they gave me that same ten-day Progesterone pill dosage I had taken before. On the third day of that cycle, I had blood work done. Then, fourteen to sixteen days into the cycle, they did another set of blood tests. Also, during this time frame, they did an ultrasound. This was to see how many follicles, or eggs, were in the ovaries and the size of each. They could also look at the thickness of my uterine lining and the size of my uterus. With this testing, they were able to find out my egg count, the average amount of eggs dropping per cycle and how the ovaries were reacting to this. They did it twice to watch the activity of both ovaries. The timing of all of this was challenging. As mentioned before, crossing the line from accepting you might need help to being ready to see a doctor is a big step. Once crossed, though, you are ready to get started. All the patience you had is now gone, and suddenly you are nothing but ready. As everything in this journey goes, though, it is a waiting game. A hurry up and wait type of situation. This means that even though I was receiving some answers, it was not quick enough.

Between all of the "womanly" side of this, they were trying to check with Michael. With the sperm, they are checking the obvious, motility and count. Beyond this, they do what is called a Kruger test. What this test does is measure the tail, head, and body of each sperm. No man has perfect results; however, you are expected to have a certain percentage of good sperm. In order to test the men, it's a little awkward. There is a cup for him to... fill... at home. Since men regenerate sperm, there is a certain timeframe in which they need to make their deposit. Then, once done, they have to turn it in within two hours.

As you can see, all of this is time-consuming and frustrating. Nothing is immediate, and your schedule has to be flexible. As mentioned in the very beginning, I was lucky. Lucky that my schedule was flexible enough that I could do all these tests. Each time I would complete a test, I would hop online and see what the results were. I wanted to know where I stood and what was going on. But I really didn't know what the test results meant. It all sounded confusing. But really, I was afraid to hear or know what was happening. I was starting out so uneducated, meaning I didn't know what the road would even look like. What if I were to hear the worst? What would the worst mean? What would Michael think? It's hard. It's like the outcome adds to the weight of waiting.

Chapter 12

There I waited, though. Through months of testing and prodding and poking and blood draws. I consumed my life with work and Roxy. I constantly tried to distract myself. But infertility consumed my every thought. I was obsessed with each test result and would try to get online and find the answers. I would guess the worst, then assume the best.

At the same time, I was becoming close with a friend we'll call Stephanie. Stephanie and her husband got married at an older age, so they were facing the natural challenges of having a child. Just because she was facing a more expected route didn't make her challenges any harder or less frustrating. Having her going through all of it with me was helpful. Misery really does love company. I would not wish the stress, energy, efforts and tears that come with infertility on anyone, but since Stephanie was struggling just like me, it was nice to know I had a companion. Looking back now, I can't remember if I was a few weeks ahead of her in the process or a few weeks behind. Either way, we were close in timing.

Stephanie and I would go on walks together around Lake Miramar and talk about our struggles and fears for the future. We shared where we were at in the process and what our plans were if things were to go south. We shared spiritual thoughts and helpful words. I will not speak for Stephanie, but for me, it was needed. Each time I saw her face smile or heard her share her positive energy with others, it brought me hope.

Hope for a happy future. Hope that everything was somehow going to work out. Hope that the future would have a happy ending. Just knowing that she was facing the same struggles, but had positive energy, was everything I needed to get through my hard times.

After a couple of months of testing and waiting, I finally got my results.

The doctor sat me down in a room with a whiteboard. He started to draw and explained to me that despite my young age, I had very few eggs left. He also said that the eggs I had left were not great quality eggs. Based on my cycle history, he suggested that there may have been times when I did not drop any eggs because the amount was so low. Both ovaries showed similar results.

He was so nice about it. I did cry halfway through his spiel, and he felt so bad that he had forgotten to bring in the tissues. He let me cry for as long as I wanted to. I remember sitting in this room all alone hearing these results. Even though he was kind, he was my doctor not my friend or my spouse. I felt cold and alone and scared. Empty.

The results were a shock.

There were no answers as to what had caused it. It could be genetic. It could be caused by diabetes. It could be because I was so close to dying that my body just attacked myself. There is no way of telling. As a Type A, crazy lady control freak, this was the most challenging part. I have played out in my mind over and over and over again, what I could have done differently in my life to prevent this infertility state. Maybe if I would have recognized my irregular periods when I was young. Maybe if I noticed that I was the last of my friends to start a real period. Maybe if I had gone to the doctor sooner when I first had symptoms of diabetes. Maybe…

Maybe I was just meant to be infertile. Maybe my body was made without the ability to produce a proper amount of good eggs, and I was meant to fight this battle. A battle full of tears and heartache. Maybe…

You can't say maybe though. You have to just take life as it is and accept these life-changing walls that we are faced with. It doesn't mean you don't fight. It doesn't mean you give up. But it means you can't turn the other way and hope for a different answer. You have to forget the maybe, take a deep breath and do what you can to get past it. Get through it. Find a way to the other side.

Sitting in the room with that doctor was when I really saw that wall. When all my fears and worries were coming to life. There were no longer any what-ifs — it was fact. I couldn't have a baby on my own. There was no "whoopsie" up ahead in my future. No way of just relaxing and letting things happen. It was hard to hear. It was hard to accept. In fact, sometimes, I still feel I have not fully accepted it. I sometimes think that maybe the doctors are wrong. Over and over again, I am faced with a daunting reality that was given to me on that day. My body does not function properly. I need medical help to have a baby.

After some tears, a nice pat on the back and a deep breath, the doctor started to tell me my options. He started out by saying that none of the options had a high percentage of results for me. However, he wanted to give them to me so that I could decide what I wanted to spend my money on, and so Michael and I could decide what we'd be willing to try.

Option 1: I would take a drug called Clomid. This is a hormone that helps your body create a lot of eggs in one cycle. So, when the eggs are dropped, there are more of them and a higher chance of a sperm finding an egg.

Option 2: IUI. This is that same procedure they were talking about trying before we moved.

Option 3: IVF. This is when you put the sperm and the egg together in a little test tube outside of the body. Once the fetus has formed to show promises of being a healthy baby, it is returned back to the woman's uterus, and all fingers are crossed that it grows for nine months and out pops a baby.

Let's talk about cost. Again, we were extremely lucky. We had crazy good insurance that covered all of these things. However, MOST are not this lucky. I would guess that about 90% of couples facing this same struggle are not covered by insurance, key word there, guess — I am not actually sure. This is a mistake. No person should have to struggle to come up with the money needed to cover these procedures. No one. People who want a baby so bad they are willing to fight their way through this should not have the extra stress of suddenly being told you can't afford it. How disgraceful is that? I have known so many women who are completely stopped in their path because coming up with the money is impossible.

The cost for Option 1 without insurance is up to $1,000. Easy. Option 2 costs more than $5,000 without insurance, and that is minus the medication. Option 3 is at least $20,000 without medication. The cost of medication varies. Depending on what exactly is needed and how much, it can be up to an additional $10,000. This is real guys. This is any little measure of hope you have just thrown out the window because that kind of money is unreal.

It's not just about raising the money, either. It's about risk. Let's say I stop eating out and take not even one vacation for a couple of years. I might have that kind of money. But what happens when I spend the money, and the procedure doesn't work? Was it worth it? Half of you are thinking yes and the other half are thinking no. For most of us suffering from infertility, we battle with both answers. Some days it is worth it and other times not. I know some of you are thinking that it seems absurd that a person wouldn't just save up money and do this. Am I not sitting here and sharing all the heartache that comes with infertility? Why would I not just sacrifice everything and save up? It's not that easy though. For the longest time, we had such a small amount of excess each month that saving up to $30,000 would take years and years and years of sacrifice. It was just unrealistic. There are also other trials with trying to save for years. Things could come up in your life where you have to spend the money you save. The procedure might increase in cost. Your doctor could retire, and in some forms, you have to start all over again. You may need to take hormone medication to help you while you wait to get money. It's not easy. There are some loan options, which really is the most ideal, but those are never a guarantee. Obviously, credit is important, but getting a medical loan is hard. Not very many banks out there give out money for making babies. It's not like buying a car that they can take back if payments aren't made. They too are risking a lot to give you money. I can't emphasize enough how much money can become the biggest stumbling block in infertility.

Going back to my situation at the time, I had three choices placed in front of me. Michael and I talked, and it seemed like option #2, IUI, was our best one. I called my doctor, and we got started.

The first step was the medication. He told me it would all be at the pharmacy. He didn't tell me that it was about three grocery bags worth of medication that all had to fit in my fridge. For the pre-procedure I had to inject some hormones. I had two vials; one had a liquid and the other had a powder. I would fill a needle with the liquid, squirt it into the vial with the powder, mix it all up then refill the needle and inject it into my stomach. This had to be done at the same exact time every night. If I remember correctly I had to give myself two shots every night. This meant four vials a night.

The next step was getting bloodwork done every three days, which meant I'd go to the hospital at seven A.M. It had to be at this time just based on timing from the medication and the timeframe of the hospital.

After a week of this medication, I went to the doctor to get a check, where they checked for the amount of eggs I was making in each ovary and the quality of the eggs. First week I had nothing. Not one egg. The doctor said he thought that might happen. Increased me to the absolute maximum amount of medicine he could give and gave it another week.

Injecting hormones into your body is unreal. It does things that are in women's nightmares. For one, it makes you very bloated. I felt like a walking balloon. Also, it makes you crazy. Think of how you are with PMS then multiply it by what seems like a thousand and bam, that's where I was at. I'm already not one of those easy going people; I already snap very easily. So, adding on these extra hormones was just a huge problem. I kept telling myself it wasn't forever. It just was a rough couple of weeks. Adding to it the nerves of everything was the lethal ingredient of making my life hell.

I got through it. We normally do get through it, don't we?

On the other side is the story told at the beginning of this story. I went in and found out after two weeks and the max amount of medicine I only created one bad follicle. That's it. I still relive this horrible moment in my head a lot — a memory that just swirls through my mind to act as a black cloud over any dreams I had had for my future. My white picket fence and beautiful house full of children has slowly become a distant dream. It takes a lot for me to believe I have that in my future. Instead, it's taken over by other things that are now my reality. The reality that children just aren't my future.

Chapter 13

After some time and thought on my situation it felt in my fate or my destiny to try infertility acupuncture. I'll tell you why I came to this decision. Remember my friend, Stephanie, that I told you about? I was talking with her and her husband about my bad eggs the doctor had discovered and what steps we were doing to overcome it. Her husband said that he has a friend who is a doctor and says no egg is actually bad. It just might be the quality of the cycle. His friend said that infertility acupuncture is generally pretty successful to help with egg "quality". I do believe in alternative medicines; I don't think they're the only answer nor always the best answer, but I do think that, when paired with conventional medical care, it's a good option to get results. So, I decided to try it.

Michael had one of those flex spending accounts through his work. For those that aren't familiar with it, I'll explain. At the beginning of the year a card is given to you attached to an account with a sum of money of your choosing. Obviously within reason. Then, monthly a certain amount is taken out of your paycheck or paychecks to pay back the sum in full by the end of the year. It's a great option when you are looking to get a medical procedure done but won't have the money upfront or time to save. In our case it was perfect because acupuncture is not covered by insurance. We decided on a total spending amount of $3,000. We felt three months, the quote given to us was $1,000 a month, was a good chance to give it a good shot.

I did a lot of research when choosing the right acupuncturist. I wanted to find one that was specifically for infertility. After some internet searches I landed on a lady who had great reviews and great results. So many people had commented on how they got pregnant after doing acupuncture with her. She was also in a convenient location, how could I go wrong? I'll never forget the small picture of the map of the area her office was at. With the freeways and streets it looked like a uterus and her office was right in the middle of it. Seemed like a sign.

My first appointment was a consultation. Honestly, it felt more like a therapy session. I was the only one in the building. She brought me back to a room that had candles and soft music, a waterfall, and comfy couches. The hallway to the office and the office itself was plastered with baby pictures and baby announcements. It felt promising. She started by asking the questions that you would expect: what's your medical history, family medical history, husband's medical history,... Then she started to ask some more personal questions. She asked me about my childhood and some childhood experiences. We focused on some items a little more than others. She took a lot of notes and was a very good listener. I felt comfortable and relaxed and that I was headed in the right direction. She said that, based on some childhood experiences, she would recommend therapy to go alongside my acupuncture. She explained that sometimes our bodies are controlled more by the mind then we realize. I agreed with her and we set up our first appointment.

Before the first appointment, again, Michael and I had to get all of our blood work and his sperm checked again. She wanted to see things as they were in that moment. Not as they were about four months earlier. Men, especially, have changed results from time to time. My results were about the same. Michael's had improved but overall it was the same. It was all good timing because I had just started my period and she was glad she could track it. I did decide to heed her advice and I also booked an appointment with a counselor before my first appointment with her. I thought a couple of sessions couldn't hurt and worth a shot.

Before I really go into acupuncture, I will share my counseling experience, because I only did three sessions. The reason I only did three sessions is because it was $100 a session and with my crazy work schedule it was hard to find time. I sincerely did enjoy it, though, and would recommend therapy to anyone in the world. Everyone has something they need to get off their chest and work through, even if they don't know it. I know because that is what happened to me.

I booked the appointment because of some experiences from childhood. Nothing crazy, but also nothing I want to go into. Just things like having divorced parents, my parents' boyfriends and girlfriends; stuff that isn't as important anymore, but I needed to talk about. During my first session, within ten to fifteen minutes, we got through a lot of stuff I just needed to say out loud to someone who knows nothing about me or my family or my life. Then, since she is a trained professional, my counselor started probing more about stress. I will never forget when she asked me on a scale from one to ten on a daily basis how stressed I was. I said, with a straight face, well I'm just like everyone else; I am usually an eight or nine on a daily basis. Her eyes kind of got big and she asked if I'm ever below an eight. I told her no, I was pretty normal. She then spent thirty minutes working with me and helping me understand that "normal" people aren't that stressed all the time. We all have moments of high stress and that's good. However, the amount I was on that high of a stress level was abnormal and we needed to work through it. For the next two sessions, that is exactly what we did. I learned that a lot of my stress came from work ,but also a great deal came from a relationship with a person in my life. Ironically the harder of the two to deal with was the work. Being a restaurant manager for a very busy and famous bakery-cafe is stressful. There is no way around it (so I thought). This meant I dealt with the personal relationship first and started to slowly cut them out of my life and create boundaries. The counselor helped me with work by giving me breathing exercises I can do at work to help me get through the day. I still do these breathing exercises to this day and am happy to say my daily stress level nowadays is around a two or three. It still can shoot up to nine, but that is rare.

I was happy I did that counseling. I did eventually get back and worked through a lot of what we started to focus on in those first three sessions. However, going back didn't happen until years and years later. Until then, stress management is something that I had to learn on my own, through use of self-help books and work with a friend who has been on a search for happiness who also studied a lot of info. I also talked and worked with my mother-in-law, who was also a trained counselor. Stress is a big deal. It controls your life more than I thought. It totally and completely consumed me. I was constantly having anxiety attacks because of the amount of stress I was having. I don't know if I would have ever known to focus on this part of me and improve this part of me if it wasn't for that counseling experience. It really helped me consider my options and look at my life and try to see ways I needed to reduce that stress.

Now, back to the acupuncture. Based on our test results, the acupuncturist, who we'll call Jan for ease (acupuncturist is a long word), recommended some vitamin supplements. They were more to help me, but she said that Michael would benefit from them as well, just because they were vitamins. Michael did notice a difference right away. He just overall felt better. I didn't really notice a difference in anything, but Jan said that was normal. These pills were very expensive. Again, insurance doesn't cover any of this treatment, so it was more out of pocket money that we just had to pay — not even using the flex account.

The actual acupuncture sessions were amazing. I would lay down on a bed. Jan would roll up my pants and my sleeves. She would talk to me about my day or my last counseling session, just whatever was on my mind, and start to put the needles in me. The needles really feel like nothing; sometimes it's a little bite but never ever really hurt. She stuck them in my feet, legs, arms, hands, neck and head. She would then turn up the relaxing music, turn down the lights and leave for a half hour. I would lay there and feel more relaxed than I ever had. I could feel the needles creating an energy in me that would flow. I could feel my body relaxing and working all at the same time. The feeling was totally unreal. I would hate when my thirty minutes would end. But, like all things, the sessions did have to come to an end. I would do this three times a week on top of home meditation and the supplements I had previously mentioned.

The first month nothing really special happened. No surprise. The second month I was so surprised that I could feel my period coming. I felt the cramps and the moodiness and hormones trying to kill me and everything in their path; you know, like PMS does. I was amazed because I couldn't remember the last time I had a period two months in a row without help from medication. Jan felt excited too and was excited to move on to some next steps. However, the month came and went, and the period never came. Jan realized she had to try a different approach. So, we decided to focus on diet in addition to acupuncture.

Since I am a diabetic, I can say that I know how much food affects you. Not just because my body doesn't process carbs and I know that it just turns into sugar that slowly kills me. It's because all foods affect diabetics. Fats make you process carbs slower. Protein "holds" insulin in your body for a little longer. So even though, technically, I can kind of eat whatever I want as long as I replace it with insulin, doesn't mean my life will always be easy and steady. This means I had to change my diet. By doing this I saw how much my body is affected by different foods. This meant that I was all for Jan's diet idea. Well, hell, I was willing to try anything to get me pregnant. Michael had to participate in the diet as well and I was relieved to hear that he, too, was willing to give it a try.

The diet was an elimination diet. We could not eat soy, corn, gluten, dairy, sugar (real or fake), red meat and I could have sworn something else for three weeks. If one meal we let one thing slip we had to start the whole three weeks over again. The night before we started I made a huge meatloaf dinner complete with apple pie for dessert. It was like a last supper. Then started three weeks of hell. You know what makes this diet hard? Well, besides the fact that it seems like there is NOTHING you can eat, you have to eat the same thing over and over and over again. Salad with vinegar or lemons for dressing. That's it. I remember when I was going through this at the same time I was working with a girl who was trying to lose weight for a bodybuilding competition so we were pretty much eating the same food. It helped me knowing that Michael and this random girl from work were struggling like me. I also often reminded myself that even one sip of soda or one bite of a cookie meant three more weeks of not eating. The third week was the easiest of the three. The cravings stopped. It became easier to find things to eat. I got used to the food and how to order. I also discovered a restaurant that had large servings of food that fit in my diet. I ate there, like, almost every day.

We made it, though. After three weeks on the diet from hell, I lost a little weight and generally felt good. We were hoping to have made some progress, however, my period still didn't start. Jan assured me that was ok. Sometimes it takes time. After the three weeks, Jan said that this is when the trial really began. What we had to do was eat the same, except for once a day, introduce one of the things we eliminated, like cheese, back into our diets in one meal. We had to do that for a week and record how we felt. Then do a week back to the diet. Then, pick a new ingredient, like corn, to do the same thing. See if anything affects us. This is how you discover if you have a food intolerance that may be affecting your body. I wanted to cry. Not only did the diet prove to be challenging because of the food we couldn't eat, but we never really had enough energy to work out, and I was eating a lot less carbs, which can be equally bad for a diabetic as it makes it hard for me to control my blood sugars. I just couldn't imagine going another three thousand weeks on this diet just to see if cheese is affecting my periods and eggs. Even typing this, that sounds ludicrous. There may be some very serious science behind that, but it made me see that this diet wasn't the answer. This direction wasn't the answer.

Right after this appointment, Michael and I were headed to LA to go see a Clippers game. That night I ate a pizza at Staples Center. It was really good. However, that was a mistake. Suddenly packing my body with cheese and carbs was horrible. I was very sick the rest of the night. Maybe, okay, probably, I should have still slowly introduced food back into my diet and not shove the greasiest form of food in my mouth in one sitting. It was equally me letting go and gaining control all at the same time. I just didn't realize this at the time. I thought I was just making a choice. A choice to eat pizza because the elimination diet was absolutely nuts. However, it was a choice to really decide where I was at in my infertility journey.

The end of this diet was also close to the time that the three months we had chosen to dedicate to this treatment was coming to an end. We had totally used all money from our flex fund plus all the extra money we spent on vitamins and expensive food. I was trying to decide what to do. I don't remember exactly what the cost per treatment was, but I know it was a lot and I would need to sustain three a week. It would have dried us out every month, plus, we would have to make some serious budget cuts. It just wasn't realistic in our financial situation at the time.

This is another example of how hard it is to make these financial decisions. I could continue to drain my wallet and my bank account. I could continue to try a procedure that had proven results. I could continue to make my schedule crazy and fit in these appointments. It would be a great sacrifice. Am I not dying for a baby? Am I not upset I don't have one? This could work. It could. Could. Where do I draw the line? How do I decide?

I was at work soon after this diet ended, and I was thinking about having to make this decision. I was standing at what we called the expo counter. Ironically I was standing there with the same girl who did the same type of diet with me while she was getting ready for her bodybuilding competition. She is such a sweet girl. She is younger than me by quite a few years, but someone that I felt was on my same level. She seemed to understand my want and need to be a mother. She was there to help me, to love me, and to motivate me. We were standing at the expo counter and chatting. I told her I decided to not continue on the crazy diet and I was considering stopping the acupuncture. She was encouraging and told me not to give up. She then told me about someone she knew that tried some diet and got pregnant. I want to reinforce that she was trying to be nice. What she didn't know is that she was the third or maybe fourth person to tell me about some diet that helps women get pregnant. For some reason, this final story of how some crazy diet helped some woman get pregnant was the end for me. It was the moment I decided that no diet or amount of money was going to get me what I was searching for. I can't continue to put energy and effort into this. It was time to let go and move on. Michael had left the decision up to me, so I knew I had his support.

To further explain, I will tell you about a diet that I remember very specifically that someone told me helped them get pregnant. They were having a little bit of a struggle and she had read something or heard something and ate only carrots and apples and got pregnant. It is true that food affects our body. I agree that if we eat right and get our bodies on the right path, we will feel better and function better. However, with me, my ovaries shut down because my body had attacked them years before; impossible to say when. Also, as a diabetic, I have to be really careful about what I am eating and how. The diet Jan put us on is similar to keto. There is science showing the dangers of putting a Type 1 Diabetic on a keto diet. We aren't Type 2 Diabetes. We are different and function different, we have to have some carbs and some sugar. So, it may be great that your sister's friend's dog walker's aunt got pregnant by drinking 1 cup of broth while standing on her head for 2 minutes every Tuesday and Thursday. That doesn't mean it's what got her pregnant. Beyond that, it doesn't even mean it's right for me. Also, it reminds me that I can never just go on some crazy diet and be lucky enough to get pregnant. If only it were that easy.

I called Jan soon after deciding I was done. She was upset. Not in a mean way, or in a way that implied that she was searching for more money out of me. She stated that I was too young to be infertile. I was too young to stop trying. She was sweet and understanding. She was loving and encouraging. I considered for a little time during our conversation that maybe I should change my mind. Maybe I should keep trying. Maybe it would be worth the money. Then she said something that stood out to me. She said, "You can't give up hope."

That's when I realized that no matter what I will never give up hope. Just because I'm stepping away from this unrelenting process of infertility treatment doesn't mean I'm giving up hope. There will always be a hope inside of me. A hope of being pregnant. A hope of being a mom. A hope that there is a light at the end of the tunnel. Hope is all I have. Even if that hope is a small light in a dark cave that is hard to see and hard to get to, it's there. It's inside of me holding me up. Getting me out of bed in the morning. Facing each day. Hope. I will always have hope.

Chapter 14

This was really a life changing decision. I wasn't just about stopping acupuncture. It was, as stated, walking away from infertility treatment for a time. Putting that life behind me and not knowing what was in the future. I had no plan. Michael and I had two options left. We could either do egg donation IVF or we could adopt. Egg donation was a hard pill for me to swallow. I can't pinpoint why. Something about the idea of seeing my husband's DNA mixed with another woman's and not mine was tough to think about. It still is, from time to time. I always thought his reddish hair, blue eyes, white eyebrows and pink skin would mix with my hazel eyes (that turn green when I'm mad), brown hair, and darker complexion. I thought together we would make the most beautiful children in the world. It was challenging for me to face this idea for lots of reasons. Mainly, facing the idea that I would have to use another woman's egg was facing that my child will never have my DNA. That's hard to handle. It's such a hard pill to swallow.

This leaves the other option of adoption. Adoption is so expensive, especially in the "great" state of California. On top of it there are so many layers and rules and experiences that come with it. You never know when the journey is going to end and you never know...really anything. It didn't seem like the right timing for us. Not being able to commit to either idea, we were left in a state of limbo.

Right before all of this acupuncture and stuff, work got intense. My current General Manager — GM for short — left on a trip to Ireland or Scotland or somewhere. She came back and just wasn't ready to face life or something. She just, like, kind of disappeared, and one thing led to another, and I became GM. Becoming a general manager of this bakery cafe chain was like all I had ever hoped for. Why, you ask? I don't even have a kind of idea. It was a huge step on my career path and a major achievement. I am happy I became a GM. I learned so much about restaurant management and everything you should not do when running a restaurant. There's no better way to learn than by making every mistake possible. It was a great place to make mistakes, because the concept is almost impossible to manage. It takes someone who is okay with letting things go, okay with some mistakes here and there, and accepting that life can't and will never be perfect. I do think and actually know there are people like this in the world. People who can handle the never-ending chaos that this bakery-cafe is. It just wasn't me.

The first month in this job I experienced stress like I never had. I often had my huge anxiety attacks where I would yell at everyone in my path and throw a fit. It's almost embarrassing to look back on. Employees were afraid to approach me and my managers didn't know how to handle me. It took me a while to get used to this new life. Since we baked our own bread, it was like I was on for 24 hours. There were managers to take care of the bakers, and even though they weren't really technically my employees, I was still responsible for them and the product they had and the items they pumped out. I was responsible for making sure everything was perfect. I just was always at work. Always. There was never a moment of no stress or any break.

I actually remember a moment when I realized work was too much in my personal life. Michael and I used to have some pretty awesome Christmas traditions. One favorite is when we get our Christmas tree.

We may have been the only Hardy's left doing this, but we loved a real tree. I used to wish we could hike into the woods, waist deep in snow with an ax, and chop down our own tree. In California — let me correct myself — in Southern California, there is no snow that is a short drive away to get a tree. What we settled on was going to a Christmas tree farm with our two dogs and getting a tree. On our way home we would stop and get some hot chocolate then put up our tree while watching The Nightmare Before Christmas. I loved this tradition. I can't pinpoint what it is about this tradition that is so close to my heart and brought me such joy. I just loved it. This one year I was a General Manager at this bakery-cafe and it was Christmas time. Michael and I were in the middle of this great tradition when my phone started going off. An employee that we relied too much on was calling out from work for the following day. It was going to ruin us. Such a busy time and a busy day. What was I going to do? I started shooting off some texts, trying to fix the situation. After one text I looked up and saw Michael looking at me with this look in his eyes I couldn't describe. He asked me something like if I was just going to work all night. I put my phone down but the moment was gone. I would never ever get that moment back. I would never be able to decide that my family was more important than my job. I think, though, this job consumed me so much it was the most important thing to me. It was me.

Earlier ,I had mentioned that I did some therapy sessions and realized I was very stressed, and it was abnormal and unhealthy. From that moment on, I started to separate myself from this idea that I needed to be a GM of this place. It was a small seed that was planted in my mind. It's something I often thought about but tried to leave behind. The seed just grew and grew and grew. I knew I needed to get away from this job. I just didn't know how.

It was mid-March of 2014 when I decided to stop doing acupuncture. Well, to stop treatments. Nine months into the most stressful job of my life. I didn't really realize it at the time, but my life was starting to fall apart. Not my marriage or anything, but me and my happiness. Without direction on what we were going to do with this infertility, I was so lost. I didn't know who to talk to because I didn't know what I needed to talk about. Work became so overwhelming and I struggled to find happiness at work, which is important. I look back at this and see and recognize the depression. During the moment, however, it was very unrecognizable. It was just a fog.

I started to get to a point where I didn't care much about anything. I was just in almost survival mode. I can't believe, looking back, that I didn't realize how sad and depressed I was. I just thought... I don't know what I thought. I just was moving day by day.

The only really good thing I remember during this time is when we got our second dog, Douglas. Anyone out there who has a lab knows how amazing they are to have. They are like built in security dogs and already know how to sense and take away your frustrations and anxiety. As I start to share the next part of my life with you, just know I wouldn't have been able to make it without Douglas. That sounds really cheesy, but it's true. His sweet demeanor and want to take care of me was there when no one else knew I needed it. He was just like Roxy. He filled a hole in my heart that I didn't even fully realize I had.

Around this time, work was struggling, just because we were becoming so swamped with catering and business of the cafe that it was hard to keep up. I found myself working mainly in catering because it was a very important part of the business and where I enjoyed being the most. I had two employees that were in charge of our catering team, Lexy & Jim. Lexy took a week of PTO and just happened to fall on one of our busiest catering weeks. This gave me the opportunity to work one on one with Jim. Jim was so fun. You know those people that are laid back about everything? They let life roll off their back and just enjoy life? That is Jim. Seriously loved working with the guy for the week. It was also nice because it gave me the opportunity to get to know him on a more personal level. I have always liked getting to know the personal side of my employees. It helps me understand them, and from that, I can be a better boss.

Our topical conversations of whatever turned into him revealing more about his personal life and what he was going through.

What I found out is that he was dating this girl for a while. They moved in together and things were going well. But, as couples often do, they decided to break up. Soon after the breakup they realized that she was pregnant. She hid it from him for a while but he was sure she was. He wasn't sure what to do. He was young, she was young. They were planning on breaking up. What do you do? I just let him talk and get it all off his chest. I was his boss and I didn't want to cross any boundaries in regards to my thoughts on the situation.

Towards the end of the week, I decided to just be honest with him. I told him that he needed to be a man. He needed to take responsibility for this child and help this poor girl take care of herself and the situation. I let him know this was his problem, too, and he needed to approach it head on.

This blunter conversation led to him being even more blunt with me about details of his situation. He told me that this girl he was talking about was another one of my employees, Julie. A few months earlier Julie had totally and completely stopped coming to work. This was totally out of character for her. She was our most reliable and best employees. In fact, when she stopped coming to work, we almost crashed and burned. When I finally got a hold of her, all she said is that she was having health problems, so she was scared and needed the time off. Since she was one of the best and she had done so much for us so many times, I told her that she should take care of herself and come back to work when she is ready.

Jim telling me that Julie was the girl that he had gotten pregnant made it all come together for me. I felt so bad for them. They were both just kids. She was only nineteen and was terrified to tell her parents. He was not much older and was also terrified of telling his parents. They just didn't know what to do. I told him I was here for them and however I could help to just let me know.

I bring you back to the present — right now. Out of my whole story that has happened, I believe this is the most traumatizing part. Just typing the line, "...however I could help to just let me know" and knowing what comes next is hard to think about. When writing this whole story out, there have been times when I have had to stop for days and weeks at a time. Reliving some feelings and experiences has been overwhelming and emotional. Each time I wrote it felt like intense journaling. Writing about this experience is different. I know the steps my life has taken. I know what was coming next. I knew this story would start and I would have to tell it. I rewrote so many parts in my head over and over again. Realizing there is no way to tell exactly what happened, or what I went through and how I felt. I have equally been anxious to get past this and just write it as I have felt anxious and not want to relive it at all. It's scary to think about. It's hard to remember. It's hard to relive. However, it's important for me to share so you can know who I am; to share so people understand the reality of infertility and all aspects and avenues; to show that not every option is the answer and sometimes all answers drag you through hell.

Back to the story…

I had told Jim I was there for him and Julie. I meant it. I checked up on him a few days after our talk about him needing to be a man and take care of the situation. He told me they talked and decided to give their child up for adoption. Hearing these words pretty much stopped me in my tracks. Adoption? Had fate just crossed my path? Did I work with Jim all week to bond with him and learn his story because this baby was meant for me? It felt like fate. I brought an idea to Michael. After we talked, I decided to do a very risky and scary thing. I told Jim that my husband and I were unable to have children, and that we have longed for a child and had often come up short. I shared with him our story. I told him that if he felt comfortable with it we would love to adopt this child.

Just a few days later I was woken around seven AM from a text from Jim. He said that him and Julie had talked, and they wanted my husband and I to know that they wanted to give us their baby.

This morning is often played out in my head over and over again. The joy haunts me and I wonder to myself if I will ever feel it again. I shook awake Michael. I told him to get up; that Julie and Jim were giving us their baby. They were giving us our baby. I cried. I found out it was a boy. Of course it was a boy. I always felt our first would be a boy. Our baby was finally going to come home. We called everyone in the family. We all cried together and we all were getting ready for what was ahead. It was a morning filled with joy. A morning that created a feeling that filled the hole that had been left in my heart over the years of unsuccessful infertility treatment. Finally, for the first time in a long time, I felt I was reaching the light at the end of the tunnel. I was going to be a mom.

This was April. The baby was due in June or July (can't remember exactly).

The steps that go into adoption are crazy. You have to have a lawyer. You have to get your home inspected. The couple having the baby has to have a social worker. You are required to pay for therapy for the birth mother. You are in charge of all hospital and medical bills that the birth mother has. Getting maternity leave is hard. You have to have a letter from your lawyer and fill out a couple extra forms. You don't get as long because you aren't actually recovering from anything. You have to decide if it's really for you. You have to do all of this kind of simultaneously, too. For us, it felt like a whirlwind.

Michael and I started with the very first step. We had to know what it was exactly we were getting into. We talked with Julie and Jim on the phone and asked them some hard questions:

Are you planning on telling your parents? Both said no.

Who in your family knows? No one in Jim's family knew. Julie's sister knew.

If your parents found out, would they try to take the baby? They both firmly said no.

Why are you giving up this baby?

That was an important question. I think for all of us. We all four had to know why we were going to come together and change each other's lives forever. They both answered that they were too young with too much in front of them. They were both scared and knew they wouldn't have family support. They wanted to provide us with unbelievable happiness by giving us something that was a source of stress and fear for them.

The conversation ended by them both assuring us this is what they wanted. They shared they were considering going down to Arizona and staying with Julie's aunt and Julie would give up the baby at the hospital. They were both positive they did not want the baby. We took a leap of faith; we trusted them.

I was scared, though — scared she would change her mind. Julie was scared too. Scared because she wasn't sure, at times, she could do it. Scared because people in her life were telling her it wasn't the right decision. However, she knew it's what she wanted to do. We knew we wanted this. We knew this was right.

Julie and I decided to create a deal. When one was feeling scared we would text the other to reassure each other everything was going to be alright. We would get through this and we would both come out on top. We would both be happier and better people. We just had to get through these two months. It worked and always helped.

Julie and I went to two doctor's appointments together. The first came with an ultrasound. Julie was so sweet. She made sure the doctor and nurses knew it was my baby. When the ultrasound happened she wanted to make sure the nurse showed me the baby. That the nurse printed off pictures for me. That I heard the heartbeat. Man what a moment. Hearing my baby's heartbeat. Seeing his little smooshed face. Knowing he was in there growing and getting ready to be my son. The son I had been waiting for and crying for; praying for and so unsure if I would ever get.

The second appointment was because they saw something in the ultrasound that seemed concerning but didn't really say what. We needed to get a second opinion. The second opinion was about as helpful as the original phone call we got about it. They just weren't sure what was going on. The doctor said there was a chance that the baby would be mentally challenged. She also said it could be nothing at all. Michael and I had decided that no matter what we were going to love this baby, so this second appointment did not change our mind. What the doctor said after I told her and Julie this was beautiful. She said that the three of us, Julie included in this, were courageous people that were doing what was right.

It felt right. Like everything in my life had led me to this moment. To get my baby.

Soon after this Julie and Jim said that the baby was ours and we should be able to experience all of the fun of having the baby and announce it to the world. I asked them so many times if they were sure. They said yes. So, the world found out that Michael and I were going to finally have a baby and he was due soon. Our friends went nuts. The love and support and excitement felt from friends from everywhere was overwhelming. I realized that more than just Michael and I were ready for us to have a baby.

I had a sister-in-law offer to throw me an online baby shower. It was very successful; we received a lot of stuff. Each package that came in the mail brought tears to my eyes. Not only because it was so sweet that all these people were thinking of us, but also because it was finally happening. I was finally, finally getting my baby. With each package the joy of setting up our nursery came with it. We had a crib and a changing table and decided to go with the theme of little woodland creatures. In the bed I set up the mattress with the sheet and a little stuffed fox. I would stare at it and imagine my little baby laying inside. Crying for me. Wanting me. Needing me. Just as much as I needed him. I imagined waking up with him in the middle of the night to care for him. I would hold him and comfort him. Tell him about the world and how he was going to make a difference. I would sometimes stare at that crib and that fox with tears in my eyes not believing this was true. I was happy we told people. It helped it feel real. It helped the fear of any ideas of losing this dream go away. It helped me know I was finally going to be a mom.

Someone that I worked with insisted on throwing me a baby shower as well. I took her up on the offer and invited all the women I knew and got ready for a baby shower. I had a good friend from the Bay Area, Mary, who really wanted to come down for the shower. I thought it was so awesome that she was going to fly all the way down to San Diego to help celebrate my long, hard dream coming true. Her coming was almost more exciting than the shower itself. That almost seemed impossible, though, because finally having a shower was unbelievable on its own.

Closer and closer the shower was approaching. I asked for the weekend off and prepared myself for a big dose of reality, I was going to have a baby.

The morning of the shower, July 21st, 2014, I was waking up a little early to get ready then go pick up Mary from the airport. We were going to go to breakfast then head to the shower. I was so excited. As I do all mornings, the first I did was grab for my phone to see what Facebook and Instagram had for me. Instead, I found some texts from Julie. My world started spinning as I was reading what she wrote.

Apparently, as the date was coming closer her sister insisted she tell her parents she was pregnant and giving the baby up for adoption. Julie was scared. She was scared her parents would disown her and scared she would never be able to talk to her dad again. In the end, she felt her sister was right, and told her parents. They reacted opposite of what she thought they would. They were excited and couldn't believe she was about to have a baby. They were very against the adoption and said she could not go through with it. She said that her mom had said I had taken advantage of Julie and her situation and that I was just there to take her baby. Julie said she locked herself in the bathroom and cried and tried to figure out what to do. What was right. In the end, she felt the only option was to keep the baby.

She was keeping the baby.

I don't know if there are words to adequately describe what I was feeling. All I could do was think of that nursery in the next room over. I thought of the sweet little onesies folded in the dresser. I thought of the little socks and shoes. I thought of the books and the blankets. I thought of his little fox sitting on his mattress in his crib. Now it belonged to no one. Now it just sat in the other room, like foreign objects in a home they no longer belonged.

She was keeping the baby.

I didn't know what to do. I didn't know how to tell people. I didn't want to tell people. I didn't want it to be real.

All I wanted to do at that moment was call Julie on the phone and talk. I wasn't mad at her. I wasn't mad at anyone. I just felt that after everything we had gone through together, the least she could do for me was talk to me. I would have told her it's ok. I would have told her that it's her baby, her choice. I would have told her that I wasn't there to take advantage of her or her situation. I honestly just wanted a baby. A baby that we had decided was mine. I wanted to tell her I was sorry if she felt differently. Sorry if I made her feel uncomfortable or pressured. I wanted to tell her everything was going to be ok. Tell her to be strong. Then to wish her the best of luck.

She wouldn't answer.

She was keeping the baby.

A baby that was never really mine but felt like mine. A baby whose sweet little ultrasound pictures were hanging on my fridge. A baby that had so many Disney clothes piled in his little dresser he was going to be dressed in style for months. A baby who I allowed myself to believe belonged to me. Who I managed to tell myself was meant to be mine. He wasn't mine at all.

She was keeping the baby.

I had to face a small part of reality and start making some phone calls. One phone call stands out to me the most. It's when I called my sister-in-law who had a brand new baby herself. I told her what happened. I could hear the baby cooing in the background. She cried for me. Up to this point I am not sure I had ever seen this sister cry. Not because she wasn't kind and wonderful and amazing, but just because she didn't cry much around people. But in that moment she cried with me. Her tears felt so comforting. Her love felt so real. Her sadness made me feel not alone. It gave me strength to get to the next call.

I honestly didn't know what to do. Mary was on a plane in the sky and I had to go pick her up from the airport soon. I had to call the host of the shower and tell her it was off.

She was keeping the baby.

Michael was mad and upset. Maybe more mad at the moment. He just couldn't understand what had happened or how it had happened. He felt helpless.

She was keeping the baby.

After a lot of useless acts and horrible phone calls it was time for me to drive to pick up Mary. Mary was one of my closest friends. I knew she would want to be there, physically there, to hold me and hug me and comfort me. However, I didn't want to tell her. Not because of any other reason then I didn't want it to be true. I had heard a lot of tears but I had not seen any but my own yet. I was afraid Mary would cry. I was afraid. How could this be happening to me?

She was keeping the baby.

Mary called just as I was pulling up to the cell phone lot. She was all giddy and excited. I instantly broke down and told her the truth. Mary was such a good friend. She offered to rent a car and drive to me. I told her I was already there and went to pick her up at the curb. When I saw her I could tell she was desperately looking at every car hoping it was mine. She wanted to get in the car and hug me. That's exactly what she did, too. She held me tight and I cried. As we started to drive away I shared the story of what happened. She just listened. It was perfect.

We decided to go straight to breakfast. We went to my favorite diner that has pancakes as big as your head. Mary was perfect during this time. She was good at taking my mind off of the subject when I became overwhelmed but equally good at talking about it when she could feel my need to talk. We decided at breakfast that we would go to Disneyland that day. We decided it was the only thing to do on a day like that.

We were right. I have been to Disneyland so many times I can't even count. It's my favorite place on Earth. This time was the best. It was everything I needed and wanted. I was still sad and still trying to figure out what I was going to do and how I was going to deal with this. At the same time, though, I was riding "Peter Pan's Flight" and "It's a Small World," catching up with my dear friend and laughing together.

After Disneyland we went more into LA and went to a Korean spa. It was relaxing. It was needed. Mary knew exactly what to do. Exactly how to make me feel better. It was perfect.

I remember the drive home from LA. It was when I first realized how the trauma was setting into my life. It had been a long and emotional day. I was exhausted, Mary was exhausted, we just wanted to be home. Mary, understandably, fell asleep. She woke up off and on to make sure I was ok and awake still. I was awake. I couldn't imagine falling asleep. I just drove in silence thinking about everything and running what had happened in my head over and over again.

She was keeping the baby.

Once we did get home, I laid in bed awake almost all night. I did fall asleep for a small portion of time, maybe an hour. I woke up and for a moment I finally felt some relief. Only because for a moment I didn't remember. But the moment left almost as soon as it had started. I had to be reminded. She was keeping the baby.

The next day we went to the San Ysidro outlet mall and shopped and shopped. We laughed and ate and had fun. That night we went to Old Town and shopped some more while stuffing our faces with Mexican food. It was a great Band-Aid. It was what I needed. I needed a distraction. I needed to not think about it. I needed to be reminded of what was good in my life.

I don't even know what I would have done if Mary wasn't flying in for that weekend. I needed her. Not just because she could get us into Disneyland for free or because she knew of a great Korean spa that she could relax in. I needed her. I needed her strong spirit and understanding of who I was and what I was going through. Every day I am grateful for that weekend with Mary. It was a bright spot in the middle of a very dark time.

Soon after this weekend I decided it was time to fly home to Idaho; to sit in a room by myself with the door locked away from the hell that was in San Diego. Michael was so supportive. He sent me on my way. He hugged me as he dropped me off. He told me to take the time I needed. He agreed to put away all the baby stuff. Michael and I have talked about this since, but I look back at this and feel like I abandoned him. That I was selfishly removing myself from a situation and making him stay in it. He said he didn't feel that way at all. He knew I needed to go and he knew he needed to stay.

That flight home was long. I had a layover in Salt Lake City then landed in Pocatello, Idaho. I tried to distract myself by watching shows on my iPad. I tried reading. Neither seemed to help the time go by faster. I cried a lot. I was alone with my thoughts. Alone with my loneliness, my emptiness. I just wanted to be home.

I was greeted at the bottom of the escalator in the Pocatello Airport by two of the sweetest faces I have ever seen, my mother and sister-in-law. They gave big hugs, made some jokes, and walked me and my stuff out to the car. I told my story. They listened. We cried. We tried to find meaning in the situation. They offered me love and comfort. I knew it was there but still felt so alone. So forgotten.

Those few days in Idaho were nice. I trapped myself in my room when I wanted to be alone and met with people when I wanted to be surrounded by love. I just didn't sleep. It was two different things. First, I couldn't stop thinking about it. That little stuffed fox on those sweet sheets in our crib just ran through my mind. I couldn't believe this was happening. I wasn't going to be a mom. Everything I had hoped for and wished for had come true and it now was all gone. The other thing was I knew if I fell asleep I would have to wake up and remind myself of the situation. That brief moment of relief would come and I would have to destroy it. It was like reliving the morning I found out over and over again. Yes, sleeping just wasn't an option.

It took about a week and a personal experience to finally get me to sleep. I remember my first real night of sleep. It was the first night sleeping at my sister-in-law's house in Rexburg. Everyone went to bed and I laid down, turned on my iPad and prepared myself for another sleepless night. It took less than 30 minutes and I was out. I slept long and hard. I woke up in amazement. I just couldn't believe I had finally slept and, upon waking up, I didn't have to relive the hell. Some sleep, real sleep, had given me the first step in moving on. See, once I started sleeping I was then able to realize my situation was real. My baby was no longer my baby. My life was taking a very sharp turn in a direction I didn't expect. I also was more willing to branch out but still only allowed the people closest to me to see me and be around me. I could tell everyone felt sorry for me but I didn't want to be reminded. Also, not everyone said the best things and it was hurtful. So, I kept my distance, saw who I wanted to and needed to see and then was forced to fly home to face my reality.

Chapter 15

People often say I recovered from that situation well. It almost makes me laugh. I don't know if I will ever recover from it. I think I will always wonder about this child and wonder if it is doing okay. I will always ache for him. I know he was never mine to have, but to me, he was mine.

Coming home from Idaho and facing my reality was horrible. The very first night I was back home my two dogs were laying on the bed. They knew I was sad and offered extra love. I laid down with them on the bed and decided in that moment that they would have to be my babies. I was lucky to have them to love me and allow me to take care of them. It was the only way I found to function and deal with the crumbling building that was my life. To this day, my dogs are still my babies. They just fill that hole and allow me to feed motherly needs I have. I don't think everyone understands the role a pet can have in your life. Dogs love their owners unconditionally. Michael used to always joke that to show who really loves you, you should lock your dog and your wife in the trunk of a car for an hour. When you come back the unconditional love of a dog will show. Obviously you can poke some holes in this theory, but the idea stands; dogs love with an amount of love that is undeniable. So, my two furry faces used their large amount of love to provide me with the caring for and taking care of that I needed. Yes, a dog can never be an actual child. However, give your friend a break when they don't have kids and choose to dress up their dog for Halloween and post it on social media. It fills a need.

To help with the transition of coming home, Michael did a really good job at putting away and hiding all of the baby stuff. That being said, I could still feel the ghosts of those items sitting in that room. I would try to avoid it and not think about it. I was never successful.

I didn't really know how to deal with any of it. The main reason behind this was that it seemed some people didn't think I had anything to recover from or deal with; specifically at work. To say that my boss was insensitive is an understatement. It almost seemed like he was annoyed by the situation more than anything. Work was just getting busier and I was underperforming because I was so distracted and spiraling.

To make the situation worse Julie had announced to all her friends that she was having the baby and it's all anyone at work could talk about. I didn't want people to know what had happened to me was because of Julie's newest news. I didn't want anyone to know it was related to my recent spiral. So I didn't tell anyone and just sat in sad silence as everyone would talk about it. The day of Julie's baby shower was a bad day for me. So often during this whole time I would hide in the freezer or office and just cry, trying to pull myself together, but couldn't. It was overwhelming and awful.

Another extra bad night at work was the day the baby was due. I wanted to take the day off but couldn't. I was closing that night and we were extra busy. I was so distracted and so sad all I could do was turn off my mind and do the best I could. There was a moment in the night when I was at my absolute lowest. I was on the brink of breaking down and trying to push through. A guest decided to overreact over a dollar. She was entitled to the dollar, and I was unable to get it to her right at that moment, and she made a huge deal that I was unwilling to get it for her. She screamed in my face. This was the straw that broke the camel's back. I started to cry. I couldn't stop it. Everyone around me thought I was a loon. The dollar Karen said that if I can't take a guest yelling at me then I was in the wrong job and walked away. I wanted to tell her what had happened. I wanted to scream to the world that a baby that was meant to be mine was due today and was no longer going to be a sweet little thing I could hold or see. I wanted so bad to explain my situation and to be hugged.

In the end I realized that it wouldn't have mattered. No one in the restaurant I was standing in and no one in the organization of the bakery-cafe I worked for was supporting me. I felt so desperate for anything that I even reached out to HR. I thought maybe she could offer some support with a direction of where to turn to get up and breathe. Her response was halfhearted, and no guidance was given. I was alone. Alone in the middle of this sea of people stuck in my sadness.

After a lot of deep thought and trying to find the best solution for me to deal with everything I was going through, I decided it was time for me to step down as a General Manager. I was not doing the cafe any benefit and, more importantly, I was not doing me any good by staying. I realized that a good option for me would be to go into catering. It's a part of the business I enjoyed and I wouldn't be taking too much of a pay cut. Honestly, it was the best option, and I was ready to be done.

I talked to my boss and told him everything I had felt and what I wanted to do. It was obvious that he did not like what I was saying. I had no idea what he thought of me as a general manager because he never gave feedback but he was fighting for me to stay. He offered some other options to see if maybe I would stay as the general manager but nothing really stood out to me. He told me to take one more weekend to think about it and get back to him. I didn't need the weekend to think about it but I did it anyway. On the following Monday I told him I wanted to step down. I told him I wanted to go into catering.

What happened after I told him this and the next big part of my story is not important. It's a lot of details where I know I was wronged and I know the situation was not handled correctly. I know my words were twisted and for whatever reason my boss took the opportunity to kick me out of this business. Maybe it's a mistake to leave out the details, but I just want to avoid a lot of "he said-she said." So, skipping ahead the next step of the story is the day the VP of the company called me at work and said he wanted to meet with me in the Clairemont office after work one day. I didn't really know what the talk was about, but I assumed he just wanted to make it clear exactly what I was wanting to do and lay out a way to reach success for all of us. I was wrong.

We sat on a big round table in a conference room. He talked to me about the way my cafe was failing and how I had been underperforming for months. He said it was a mistake to agree to adopt a baby from a former employee. He said that it might be time for me to just move on.

I tried to tell him that I had been wronged. I tried to tell him I was passionate about the brand and the franchise. I tried to tell him it wasn't time for me to leave.

He didn't listen.

He pulled out a severance check for one month and made me agree to not apply for unemployment. I wish I would have recorded the conversation so I could have applied for unemployment and won. I was wronged. The whole situation was wrong. I was being forced out because of depression. I was being forced out and even though I had reached out to HR asking for help for my spiraling life. Even though they all knew I had lost this child. Even though they had no real reason, evidence of feedback or evidence for firing me, they let me go.

Right when he pulled out the check I broke down, really broke down, for the first time. I cried like I had not cried yet. It was the lowest I had been or felt. I told him that. I told him I was lost and confused and depressed and I didn't know what I wanted to do or what I should do. Even though in the moment I wasn't that big of a fan of the man in front of me, what he said next helped shape my future and I was grateful for it.

He told me that on the previous Sunday he was preaching at church. He was teaching the story from the Bible when the disciples were out on the waters during a storm. They were scared and Christ walked on water to them to help calm the storm. He was out on the water and called Peter out to him. Peter started to walk towards Christ in faith. Then in a moment he started to get scared and started to sink. Instantly, Christ reached out his hand to pull Peter up. The VP said that this is where I was at this moment. I was starting to sink. The key word to this Bible passage is the word "instantly." He emphasized the story again, instantly Christ reached for Peter to pull him up. He told me that he had no doubt that instantly Christ was going to reach down and pull me up.

I hoped he was right. I hoped Christ was there reaching out for me to pull me up. Because there I was. Walking out of a building with no job, no child and no idea for the future. What was I going to do? How was I going to get through this? In some ways my whole life was ahead of me and this was perfect and what I needed. I needed to be let go and I needed to be forced out. In other ways I was so lost and confused and scared. It was the true end of the biggest chapter in my life. It is all still unbelievable to me how it all happened. A moment of complete darkness and forcing myself to put my foot out in front of me and trusting there was ground to step down on.

I no longer would consider myself a religious person. I have been recently introduced to the word "agnostic" and it fits me perfectly. I don't know if Christ reached down instantly when I was sinking in the water. I don't know if my life ahead was what anyone intended for me. But I do know that once the shock of that moment wore off and after I got my head on straight that I was determined to do something for me. I decided I needed to take control of my life instead of letting life control me. No more fate. Just me.

Being unemployed is hard. Especially when you are as lost as I was. I had no idea what I wanted to do but what I did know is that I didn't want to manage a restaurant ever again. The long hours, heavy stress and no weekend thing that came with managing a restaurant was a road I never wanted to take again.

So, I did all I knew I could do. I created a resume and applied for every job I could think of. I focused my energy and emails for jobs in the administrative industry. I knew I didn't have experience in these areas but I knew I could do it. I had to sell myself and it was hard. I know I was in a pool of people who were also unemployed but had experience. Also, I know I stood out to people because in a lot of applications I had to write what the pay for my previous job was and I'm sure they were wondering why I was taking a pay cut and how I was going to be okay with it. I just didn't know what to do. In the meantime, I had only four weeks of severance, so I needed to find something fast.

Anyone that has been unemployed knows this cycle well. You start out not picky but not desperate. You comb through Craigslist and Indeed with hope and a lot of options in front of you. You don't feel scared or worried you just go. Then, as time starts to move on your expectations of what you are looking for in a job change. You start to look at jobs you passed by in the past. You start to look at lower salaries. Your idea of what a good job might be changes a little bit. Then, you become desperate. You just want anything to make any type of money. Your pride is gone and you are just struggling to make things work.

For me this process took about a month to go through. I did have a good distraction. I got really into a workout plan and tried to become a millionaire through a multi-level marketing business. Obviously it didn't work, because I am not a millionaire, but it was a good distraction. Through that time I learned to focus on me and give attention to me. I was able to focus on my body and my health. In such a trying time I needed something to help make me happy and get me through my day and that did it. On top of that I was able to share my story more. Share more about me and who I am. In a month I got one thousand hits on my blog and people started to reach out to me. Women who were infertile or just barely starting to struggle or were scared they would struggle messaged me with advice and more questions on my story. I learned how to be confident in my story and confident in who I am. I mentioned before how I don't know if I believe in fate. However, I do feel finding this workout program was good timing. It gave me the confidence and boost I needed.

During this time I not only gained the confidence I needed I learned a lot about myself. As mentioned before I had it kind of embedded in my brain that I was going to be a stay at home mom. Both those influences from my family and community and the idea that it's what I had wanted. In fact, when I was first married, Michael said that he wished he could make enough that I could just be a stay at home wife, and I longed for it. Sometimes I would think that being able to stay at home and not work, sometimes, was my main motivation for wanting a baby. This idea that I would be able to stay at home, take care of my child, clean my house, run errands and make dinner seemed like a dream world. What I learned after a couple of months of being unemployed is that is the exact opposite of what I really wanted in my life. Even though being unemployed and childless is different from a stay at home mom, I suddenly realized that the thought of staying home at all was just not for me. I liked the idea of having a career. I loved the idea of growing with a company and wanting to be on the top. I loved the idea of working forty-plus hours a week and then coming home and having to juggle life. I needed my days off to be filled with errand running and house cleaning. I don't like idle time. Now, I do enjoy vegging, and I think it's important to take a day to do nothing to let your body reset. However, I don't like doing it for a full day every week. I need my days filled.

Now, before I have a mob of stay at home moms at my door, let me say this. Lots of people I know are stay at home moms. Their lives are crazy busy. Sometimes they don't even have time to respond to a text because their lives are so full. I know that this choice in a job is not one that comes with dull moments. However, it's not one where you can climb a corporate ladder. It's not one in which you get to interact with adults who have the same occupation for eight hours of the day. I need that. I didn't realize I needed it until I didn't have it. It wasn't even until the end of my unemployment that I realized it was missing from my life. I felt empty and useless. It was such a valuable and an important thing to learn.

Chapter 16

You don't really need to hear about the sad jobs I had while unemployed. Nothing exciting. I will tell you about the last job I had before getting started back on my career, though. I found a job as a server at a Chinese buffet. I made enough money (mixed with another side job I had) working seven days a week and it wasn't terrible. This restaurant had no real management system set up. It was like a "mom and pop" type place, but insanely busy. I realized after a few months of working there that I was starting to manage the servers. Nothing crazy, but just managed the situation and tried to coordinate things and interact with the hostesses. I just fell into a pattern, almost like muscle memory. It kind of caught me off guard. Once I did realize what I was doing, I realized that I was fighting a losing battle with myself. All that time I had been trying to find a job out of the restaurant industry. I was trying to escape a world of chaos and customer service. The reality? It is what I was made for. It's what I enjoyed doing and what I was good at. It came natural to me. I had learned a lot over the years and I needed to use that knowledge. Not just because I had but because I wanted to. I wanted to be successful. So, I changed my mindset.

It wasn't long until after my realization that I found a job as a manager of a sandwich chain with promises of moving up to district manager fast. Man, what a crappy job. There was not one thing I did that was criticized and wrong. Even if I was right it was wrong. My first week there my district manager went in and did my deposit for me. He found that $100 was missing and blamed me, saying I stole it. I can't believe what I had to go through to prove I never stole it. This wasn't the only time that happened. Over and over again my district and regional manager took shots at me and tried to find a reason to fire me. I did go to HR a few times. I went as high up as I could. I was just told that the regional manager gets results, so he is not changing his game. There were times when I had moments where I thought I would be able to do this long term, but they were very short lived and far apart. I knew I was doing a good job. I knew what I was doing. I knew I could make a difference if they let me. But they wouldn't let me do it.

I lasted three months at that job before I found the perfect job for me that has led me to a real start at a successful career. Three months is all it took for me to realize that I'm better than being yelled at, put down and consistently framed for stealing. I will never feel pride for my work I did at this sandwich chain. It's too bad because I had good ideas and the right skills. They just weren't interested. I'm happy this new company I applied for was ahead of me. I just knew I could make changes there.

In July of 2015 I started with a company that manages restaurants in airports throughout the world. The job was so unlike anything I had ever done before, but it was perfect. It was equally challenging and easy. It was easy in the sense I knew how to make changes, but challenging because I had to make changes. What really stood out to me was the way I was supported by my managers. I had never had a job where I was more supported than this. They saw my talent and my potential. They allowed me to do what I needed to do. I was able to move up fast and make large changes quickly. Still, as I look back my heart swells with pride for the things I did and the way I did it.

Starting my new job. really gave me purpose again. Starting there and gaining back a lot of confidence I had lost is what helped me get my head back on and start thinking about my life, where I was headed and, ultimately, my infertility journey. I finally was able to imagine myself moving on and moving forward and getting a child.

It was around this time that my mind started to get opened up to egg donation. As a reminder, egg donation IVF is where I use someone else's egg, Michael's sperm and my oven. The doctor said it would be about a 60% chance.

This mindset of refocusing back on my hormones and my body got me back to the doctor. I had been having some strange symptoms and I decided to look into it. I went to the doctor and told her my symptoms and she did not look impressed with anything I had to say. I actually honestly think she didn't believe me. But she did some tests and sent me on my way. I got a call about a week later and was told to come back in. She told me I was going through menopause. The hot flashes, tiredness and various other symptoms mixed with my test results were a sure sign of menopause. She said at my age with having such a low amount of estrogen I needed to get on birth control so I could cycle and get some estrogen back to avoid osteoporosis in my future.

I cried in the pharmacy waiting for my pills. I don't even really know why. I just didn't want to hear more of how my body wouldn't make babies. I didn't want a reminder of the ways my body was failing me and my heart. Also, I really didn't want to be on birth control. I don't care if I am told there is no chance in hell I will ever have a baby on my own. I don't want to prevent it. I wanted to hold onto these imaginary chains of hope that there was still a chance I was going to have a baby.

When you are infertile, you are told by others and by yourself to never give up hope on having a child. When I think about hope for my future, really, I think not so much about never giving up hope for having a child but more about never giving up on the idea that I will be happy and can find peace. I don't want to give up hope on my future. I do, however, want to give up hope on becoming pregnant. The hope that lives inside me that one day I will get pregnant is buried under a lot of bitterness and anger. However, it's like a beaming light in a hole of darkness; not missed, but seen and shining bright. Hope is all that people who are infertile have. However, if not handled correctly, it can be destructive.

A very well-known Bible passage is that faith, even the size of a mustard seed, can move mountains. Faith is equivalent to hope.

This hope devours me in a lot of ways. It becomes so destructive and shows its ugly face in many ways that I can catch glimpses of throughout the years. One way that hope constricts me was in the form of pregnancy tests.

The week before my period is one of the most stressful times in my life. Just think, it happens every month. I have learned to realize the psychological toll the week before a period actually takes. Already, I feel extra hormonal because of PMS. My mind becomes a lot more on edge and I'm already a high strung person. I think it's a semi cruel joke that pregnancy symptoms and period symptoms are the same. They should be clearly different. Everyone would benefit from that. Everyone. So, the week before I start I have cramps, nausea, fatigue, moodiness, sore breasts, low blood sugar... oh! and the added never ending hope that one day I might actually be pregnant. So every symptom I have leads more and more to this undying belief that I might be pregnant. I try to push away the thoughts but they are always there. This constant struggle becomes exhausting and interacts with my already-there PMS. It starts to make everything more stressful than it actually is. My mind slowly becomes unable to comprehend the easiest stuff. With work I suddenly find myself reading the same email over and over again trying to make out the words and just understand what is being asked of me. On conference calls I struggle concentrating and taking in the information. I spend my whole day on pins and needles; it's not just mental either. My muscles are all tense. Sometimes I feel my shoulders are living by my ears because the stress is so bad and my muscles so tight. To make matters worse, there is no relief. A long walk, a hard run, a good workout, a hot bath....nothing brings me the relief. It's almost like a disease spreading through my body. Multiplying and making things worse. I am just in constant battle with one side of my mind telling me over and over again that I am not pregnant and will never be pregnant so to calm down. Meanwhile the other side is telling me over and over again exactly why I am wrong for thinking that; that I am pregnant and it's okay to accept this knowledge and to let it soak into my thoughts. Both sides get louder and louder the closer the time of the actual period starts. Because my body is so tense and my work is suffering and I no longer seem to function in my own home, I tend to get migraines. Long lasting, many day migraines that are not even dulled by pain medication. Sometimes it's almost too overwhelming and I don't know what to do to stop it. I just have to live in this confused, unfocused and stressed out state for a week. Then starts what I call, the pregnancy test cycle. Over time my periods got further then and further apart then eventually stopped, however, I always found myself in the same pregnancy test cycle. This cycle, that I'm about to describe in detail, is destructive. It's very unhealthy and causes severe damage to a person mentally. That being said, this is real. This is a cycle not just experienced by me but experienced by lots of infertile women around the world. Some women never stop this cycle. Some never tell anyone that it is happening. However, it happens. It's hard, it's lonely and sometimes scary.

Here you are having all these "symptoms" and this argument with your brain when suddenly you start to really think and imagine the feeling of actually telling your husband or your friends that you're pregnant. You imagine that feeling of overwhelming joy that would overcome you and your loved ones as you cry together and rejoice in the miracle that has taken place. You imagine people telling you "This is why you never give up." It becomes so real you can actually feel it happening. You can feel the tears. The happiness. This is when hope has the most control. You get convinced that you are pregnant and buying a test is the best solution.

Have you ever gone grocery shopping on a diet and walked by your favorite cookies? You walk by. Stop. Stare. Debate. You think about how good you could be and how balanced you would make your diet. How it's okay because we need sugar and balance is good. Have you? That's what it's like standing in a drug store staring at pregnancy tests. Except worse. The moment I end up down that aisle and see the price of these stupid sticks you pee on my brain starts to reset. It starts to realize the mistakes I've made and question how I got to this point. I can tell you right now that every time I have gotten to this point, more than anything, I have just wanted to walk away. I just want to take a deep breath and accept that this never happened. I never have, though. I have always purchased the test. I grab the test and walk to the counter as a large debate starts in my head. I go between the logical side of my brain telling me there is no way I'm pregnant to the side of my head where all my friends and strangers of the world are telling me to never give up hope. That a miracle can happen at any time. To just have faith and pray. Honestly, it's almost surreal. I really don't know what side to believe and it's almost like my body goes through the motions of getting to the cash register without any control by the arguing brain that's in it. But I always purchase it. Once I have walked out the door I have this moment of full clarity and realize the mistake I made. It washes over me like a wave of water. I shamefully wrap up the bag and shove myself into the car and allow the self-hatred to take over. Hatred that I allowed myself to get this far.

Taking the test can go one of two ways; it really depends on how long the moment of clarity lasts. Usually by this point I know the test is going to be negative but sometimes there is a small beacon of hope strobing inside. If I still have this beacon of hope I will wait to take the test in the morning. It's really so I can squash that hope like a bug. It's the only way to really kill it. If the hope is already gone I take the damn thing right away just to see the negative really fast and get it over with. Notice how no matter what I still take the test? That's because even though I say there is "no hope" there absolutely, positively will always be a small amount of me that wishes my clarity I was suddenly feeling was wrong. I never fully reset to a mindset of not being able to get pregnant. Not accepting it. No matter how much hope lives in me or how I take the test I always end up holding and staring at a negative pregnancy test.

Just like you should never say never; you should never say always. There have been two times in my life where I have truly thought the damn thing was positive. Those times are worse. As an infertile woman who had just gone through a roller coaster of believing she was pregnant then immediately switching over to accepting that she is not, staring at a positive pregnancy test is confusing and not in any type of good or positive way. It honestly feels like what I imagine winning the lottery feels like. An overwhelming feeling of relief, excitement, disbelief and joy. The feeling is unstoppable for me. I am instantly overcome with happiness like I have never felt. False positives are more destructive than instant negatives. Once I realize these positives that I see are not real the fall is much harder.

This cycle is not only driven by hope in the sense that you hope to see the positive — sometimes you need to see the negative. Sometimes your imagination has the best of you, but you somehow still have control over your logic and it's like a war inside your head. It gets confusing on who to listen to and becomes overwhelming. On the one hand, you want hope to win, because you want to be pregnant. On the other side, you know logic is the safer way to go and less heartbreaking. You feel torn. Sometimes the only way to calm your brain and help straighten you out and ensure sanity to return to your life you need to see a negative. It's like your brain is in an argument about whether or not the sky is blue. Then suddenly logic pushes hope outside to show them the sky and hope suddenly can't argue anymore. The sky is blue and you can't deny it. Sometimes I need that moment I can't deny. Sometimes I need to know without a doubt that I am not pregnant. The negative is a form of comfort. However, that being said, it still brings heartache. Hope is still there looking through the same set of eyes down at a test thinking about all the good things that come with a positive result. Even with the comfort of a negative comes the heartache of it.

In the end whether I needed to see the test to calm my mind, I saw an instant negative or I saw a false positive, I am left with this same empty feeling.

As I write this today, I am ending one of these cycles. This last one was bad. I had seen one of the two positives I had talked about. I actually thought I was pregnant. When reality started to set in I crumbled. I actually wanted it all to end. Not a suicidal end but just an end. I realized it needed to be my last cycle ever. I am going to look for a counselor this week in hopes I can end this destructive cycle. It was today that I realized that the only thing that comes of all of this is self-loathing. The idea that I can allow myself to be so excited and so over the top and so willing to accept that my deep fantasies are reality is discouraging. When I'm here, at this moment, I just want to go back in time. I don't want to move forward because I don't want this moment to even happen. I want to take back the last few days. I want to leave the world and escape the foolishness I feel. I want to cry until my tears are gone and be alone. I somehow convince myself that I am alone. All alone. I feel so embarrassed and hate myself so much that I don't even want to be around my husband. However, equally. I want him to hold me and tell me it's okay. I'm okay. But it's not okay.

I'm not okay. In fact I feel quite the opposite. It's in these moments that the weight of the reality of what is wrong with me hits me the hardest. I feel so overwhelmed with hatred towards my body. I sit here and wonder "why? Why is this ok? Why must women across the world face this problem?" It then somehow morphs into wondering why I can't just get over it. Why must I define myself by having children? Why must I think that the only way I can and will be whole is by a child?

It feels like it should be so easy to know that I can't have children. To know that I will never have the moment you see on TV or hear about where you and your spouse sit and hold hands on the bathroom floor while the test sits on the counter. Then when the timer ends you grab it and hug and cry and embrace in excitement. I know this moment will never come. Yet I still yearn for the excitement. I still yearn for the moment when this will happen. I used to fantasize creative ways I would tell my family members that I was pregnant. Now I just fantasize even saying the words "I'm pregnant" at all. To shriek to the world that miracles do happen is one I long for deeply. This excitement and this idea of announcing something so joyous is what stops my logical mind from taking a back seat to my fantasy mind.

I once tried to get rid of these cycles. For work one year I spent two weeks in Denver. At the time, my dad lived outside of Denver in a town called Evergreen, and I stayed with him instead of getting a hotel. Evergreen is in the mountains. As I would drive to my father's home I would slowly become surrounded by tall trees, thick snow, and wildlife. It had been a while since I had really been in the woods surrounded by nature and wanted to take advantage of that in more ways than one. I started by buying a pregnancy test. Of course I wanted it to be positive but knew it would be negative. On my day off I peed on the stick and wept as I saw the negative. I wanted this to be the last time. I got all bundled up, wrapped up the stick in a bag, shoved it in my pocket and left to a nature hike. It was March while I was there. There was light snow and it was very cold; naturally, not a lot of people out. I hiked just a half mile into the woods and sat at a bench next to a garbage can. I sat in complete silence and looked at and enjoyed the nature around me. There was something so incredibly peaceful about the environment I was in. After sitting in silence for an unknown amount of time I told myself it was time for the pregnancy tests to end. It was time to leave the heartache of taking these damn things in the woods with the test. I told myself this was it. This was the last time. I threw away the test and walked away. I was so confident I would never test again. I felt so proud and excited for the future. Ready to start anew. I remember feeling so proud of myself and couldn't wait for my life ahead.

Just like an addict, though, it didn't take long for my inner desires to overcome the logic and part of my brain that tells me to stop when hurting myself. Like an addiction the cycle started back up and I did it silently so that no one knew. The cycle continued each time taking more and more effect on me and tearing me down inside. I was mad at myself for "falling off the wagon". I had tried so hard to stop taking tests. To end my cycle. I often thought about my trip in the woods and wondered how it had not worked. How had I not been able to stop. It wasn't until later that I realized I didn't really want to leave my pregnancy test taking addiction in the woods. What I really wanted was to leave the desire to ever see a positive one in the woods. I wanted to leave any hope I had of becoming a mother behind.

This leads into actual positive tests. What am I talking about? Oh, the people around me who actually have positive tests, because they are actually pregnant. For most infertile women, a pregnancy announcement is some of the worse news. You go through this strange cycle. First, you feel a small window of joy. Then, almost immediately after the seconds of joy, you feel overwhelming sadness. It's sadness because it's a reminder that you are not pregnant; a reminder that you have no idea when you will be pregnant, a reminder that you don't have the money to get pregnant. Then it mixes with jealousy that your friend can get pregnant. Then, you feel bad; guilty, really. Guilty that you are upset with someone for being pregnant. You should only feel joy. Why do you feel mad and jealous? What is wrong with you? It then spirals into this dark alley of self-hatred about you, your body, your state of mind and your situation. When friends have told me they are pregnant I have totally stopped talking to them for hours. I hate myself for it. I just want to be happy for them but I can't be. Not at first. I need time and I hate that.

Chapter 17

Everyone has a coping mechanism for when they are struggling with feelings. For some it's salty food, sweets, sad movies, you name it. For me it's shopping. I just feel so down, I need a pick-me-up, and clothes, shoes and makeup help me feel pretty. Once, after a friend told me she was pregnant and I knew she didn't want to be; it was a total surprise and she was worried about the future, I went out and had a very destructive shopping spree. I just couldn't deal with the emotions of it. These announcements have gotten worse over the years, too. I cringe when I'm scrolling through Instagram and see a possible pregnancy announcement heading my way. I just don't know how to react anymore. I know the root of the problem. I know why I feel the way I do. It's just part of the struggle. You have to learn to deal with it.

Months after the announcement of the actual pregnancy comes the baby shower invitation. I decided at some point that going to baby showers is just one of the unhealthiest things I can ever do for myself. I stopped going. I just can't sit there and watch presents be opened and see the joy and happiness for anyone. That sounds terrible, but it's true. It's just too overwhelming and I am just too sad after. I'm sad that I am holding onto this idea that it's supposed to be my turn and I'm tired of it being everyone else's turn. I get caught, again, in hope.

The thing is, if I'm not holding onto hope, how do I move on? I'm at such a low low at this point – between the pregnancy tests and announcements. How do I pick up the pieces and move on? The honest answer is...I don't know. I don't know how to gather up myself and get my life back on track. I guess part of it is because, what would the point be for me to sit down at the bottom and wallow? What do I gain from that? Maybe it's from years of practicing the yo-yo of infertility, and slowly as the falls have gotten harder and harder, I have adapted to dealing with myself getting back up. I don't know. What I do know is it seems harder as the years go on. Each time it happens I further have to accept the reality of the body I was given; to accept that no matter how much I want it, how hard I try to get it and whatever tricks are out there for me to try, I will never get pregnant by surprise, if pregnant at all. I don't have to be okay with this fact but I need to accept it. Accepting reality is how we live in it. It just feels impossible to do it. Life doesn't ever seem to wait for you, though. It just comes how it comes and you have to face it and decide how you want to deal with it; acceptance or further denial lost in the hands of hope.

Again, with these birth control pills, life was not waiting for me to figure my shit out. Here I was at this stage where I was at an end. Menopause is the end of having babies, right? And I hadn't even started. I was right where my life seemed to lead with every negative test and every baby announcement. A large reminder that life is not going any way I ever expected it to be. Here I was, again, feeling like I was being forced to accept this loss of hope in my life. I had to accept and move on that I will never get pregnant or…. Or what?

So, I decided to allow myself to stay shackled in the chains of hope and doing that meant that I wanted to stop taking those birth control pills I had been prescribed. I just felt there had to be a better way to get estrogen into my body without stopping any hope I had for getting pregnant. It seemed to be the same part of my brain that was involved in my pregnancy cycles or in my destructive shopping sprees with a baby announcement. I wanted to stay in this stage of hope for the future in getting pregnant.

Soon after stopping birth control, I changed insurance companies. So I could just set up care in several different places, I made an appointment with a new gynecologist. I told her my story and what I had gone through up to this point. She wanted to do a few tests just to see on her own what we were dealing with. What she found out is that I am going through "menopause," however, when you are under the age of forty, it's not normal. The normal thing is being over forty and having menopause. The abnormal thing is to be under forty and going through these changes. These symptoms for someone under the age of forty cause a condition called Premature Ovarian Failure or POF.

I'm not going to pretend that hearing I have POF was joy to my soul. What I am going to say is that having a name for my condition was relieving. Finally, I knew what was wrong felt like an answer. I had POF. I could go into doctor's offices and say I have POF and they know what I meant. I didn't have to relive and retell my story over and over again. I also could make a real plan for what I would do to get a baby.

This gynecologist really gave me a new mindset and a fresh breath of air. She will never know or understand what she did to help me. Not only did she give me this long lost hope I had been looking for by giving me a fresh breath, but she also helped me really wrap my head around egg donation. She shared with me two different women she knew personally who did egg donation IVF and how wonderful their experiences were. She encouraged me to think seriously about it. It was like in the times I was in her office I wasn't just a patient. I was someone she was really rooting for and someone she wanted to see have success. She encouraged me every time I was in there to call a fertility specialist and to get an egg and get pregnant. It's amazing how people just come into your life and cross your path without them even realizing what kind of impact they have on people.

Her encouraging words are exactly what pushed me over the edge. They were exactly what I needed to hear to help me decide that egg donation IVF is something we needed to try. Something we needed to put our efforts into and give a shot. I realized that if it worked it would be great and wonderful and amazing. If it didn't it would be everything checked off our list of possibilities and adoption would finally be a real option, and eventually, we would be able to visit that idea again. I told Michael and we took a deep breath and decided it was time to really look into it.

Please keep in mind that each person has to come to this acceptance on their own. You can't force anyone to agree to any procedure, the idea of adoption, or wanting to foster. You can't. Each person has to mentally tell themselves that a stage in the process is over and you have to move on to the next one. Sometimes this takes a long time, and your continual pressure for them to accept it and "just adopt" or "finally foster" isn't helping. In fact, it often pushes them away from accepting what they are going through. My doctor had the right approach. She assessed how I felt about the situation. She saw I was teetering towards the edge of giving in. She mentioned it once, then immediately dropped it when she heard I wasn't interested. Then she tested the waters but not in an obvious way. I was coming to her a lot, trying to find results and answers and ways to have children, and she knew this was the only way. She knew that in order to get me what I wanted, egg donation IVF checked off most of my boxes for having children. She helped me see that in a healthy way. She was never forceful and was always just suggesting. Also, since she was a professional in the field and knew what she was talking about, she approached it in that manner. Just medically. I know it seems easy to just move onto adoption or move onto IVF or go to the doctor in the whole first place but just keep in mind it's mental too. It's a deep acceptance that your body isn't normal. That you may not get what you are looking for.

On the same note of telling someone to "just adopt" or "finally foster", one thing you often hear is, "You need to or should focus on the children you do have in your life." There is this idea that I can help them and be surrounded by them and it's equally as nurturing. I spent probably a total of seven or eight years teaching the kids at my church music. It was a fun way to volunteer for my church. I love music and really did enjoy teaching them lessons through music. I felt fulfilled and happy. However, the way I felt fulfilled wasn't in the way everyone seems to expect me to. I never felt like any of the children were filling this hole I felt from not being a mother. In fact, as mentioned before, I am not very maternal and often don't really like children. So, even though I enjoyed the hour or two I would spend with these kids, it was nowhere near how I wanted to feel. The closest I feel to motherhood is with my nieces and nephews. In fact, I have a niece that is a lot like me. When her mom tells me about the struggles her daughter is going through I feel like it tugs at the strings of my heart because I get her. I get why she acts the way she does. Her mom, my ex-sister-in-law, used to reach out to me a couple of times asking for advice. That really helped. It really does. I feel like I'm passing on my wisdom and knowledge to help a tiny human become part of this world. It feels fulfilling. However, these moments are few and far between. Now, with my three best friends, I have eight children in my life that I help influence on a regular basis. Still, the moments of "mothering" are still few and far between, and not the impact I am looking for. In the end, my parenting style is too different, and in the end I will never be their mother.

I feel like I have a lot of life experience. I had to go through a lot in high school and make some hard decisions. I feel like I made a lot of the wrong decisions so I can look back and see how I would have done it differently if I would have had different guidance and something to help me get through when I didn't know what direction to go. I'm not saying I'm going to be the perfect mom, or that my children will even listen to me at all. But I want to try. I want to give advice and help them get through the hard times. This may be a little too much into the mind of a crazy person but sometimes I even practice what I would say if my daughter asks me about wanting to have sex, or what I would say to my child who wants to go to a party and start drinking, or what I would do if my kid came home and was upset about their boyfriend or girlfriend breaking up with them. I've practiced how I plan on telling my child that Santa Claus and the Easter Bunny are real but not in the way they think and how to help them understand the magic that comes with believing in them. I just want to pass on this knowledge so much that I have spent hours and hours in front of my bathroom mirror, or while I was driving to and from work, relaying pieces of my past and what I did in situations like that and what I wish I would have done instead, or what I did right and how I feel because of my decisions. This information is just passed on to what seems like a ghost.

It goes beyond wanting to teach. I want to have experiences with them. Each time I watch a Disney movie or go to Disneyland I am overwhelmed with feelings of wanting to experience those things with my child. I want to be the parent that buys them everything they see while walking down Main Street, USA. I don't want to look at the people around me but, rather, watch my child's face as they look in wonderment at the world around them. I long to kiss boo boos, make lunches, and even fight over whether or not their blanky can come with us to the store. People share these experiences in their lives and I see it through social media and I long to be in those situations. I want to feel the pride these parents show in their children. I want the joy that only comes from motherhood. It's great that I have children in my life, but they aren't mine, and they will never be mine. My love can only reach them so far and it will never feel far enough.

I know what people mean by saying the children in my life can act as placeholders for my own children but it's not the answer.

There is also, "Just come and watch mine and then you will never want kids again." I also know what people mean by this. However, this is not something you should ever say to someone struggling with infertility. I just don't want to stop wanting. I don't want to spend time with children that I don't feel some maternal bond for in hopes that by the end of the couple of hours my want for children will leave. Why would I want that? Why would I ever stop wanting?

Chapter 18

Looking into egg donation IVF helped me open my eyes into another side of infertility I had not focused as much on — Michael's side of the grief. When we first looked into egg donation IVF, we started by signing up for a company that had good reviews. They had egg donors already ready to go, facilities all throughout California and a consultation to help you answer any questions you had. During the consultation we were asked a lot of questions about us. Turns out they wanted to know about us so the egg donors felt good about giving their eggs. I thought that was a nice touch. It was the first glimpse I had into Michael's heartache. I realize it is selfish in thinking this, but I had not once thought about any heartache or struggle he was going through. He just never talked about it. If anyone out there knows Michael on any type of personal level you will understand that he just does not share feelings. However, he had to share some in order to answer this company's questions.

The first moment I realized it was during the online questionnaire when he had to put on a scale of one to ten of how much he is affected by the idea of infertility. I don't remember what number he picked but I know it was over five and suddenly a ton of bricks landed on me; he was affected. Then as he answered more questions, and when we had the actual consultation on the phone, I started to fully realize the struggle that comes with infertility for him. I was in full realization when, once, I struggled so intensely to get out of bed due to depression that I wrote down all of the things bothering me. Two of those things were: that we do not have a child yet and I don't know when we will ever get one, if we ever will. I showed Michael the list because it was the only way I knew how to tell him about what I was going through. The next day I was lying in bed, refusing to get up, and he came to talk to me. He told me everything, then emphasized the word everything, on that list are things he struggles with daily too. Then told me what he does to fight through those struggles. That was the moment I finally and totally understood that he was struggling just as much as me. Infertility affected him just in ways that were different. Michael never came to doctor appointments and learned everything secondhand through me. He then never talked about his feelings with it. So how would I know?

I once took a marriage class with Michael. Part of the class was learning about sharing problems. The teacher, a trained and successful family therapist, said that sometimes one or both members of a couple have a hard time understanding what their partner is going through. If the other spouse has a problem it can be easy to let yourself consider that their problem. However, you have to remember that in a couple, it is your problem. She said a good way to think about it is to imagine that both of you are in a room and in the middle of the room is a box. You both can approach the box, touch the box, move the box so the box belongs to both of you. It's the same with these big problems, like infertility. It's a box in the middle of the room. Both members of the couple need to remember at all times that it is their problem. The wife needs to share her struggles and her heartaches with her husband. He needs to listen and understand. No matter who has the biological problem, you both need to hold each other up and listen to each other's needs. From the beginning. I can promise you that by being honest and upfront and sharing in the beginning will save heartache in the end. Whatever that end may be.

Often the men get forgotten when it comes to infertility. We focus on the woman and her needs and her struggles. Whether it's the husband's "fault" or the wives', both grieve. Both want a family. Both long for the moments like when the water breaks, when the baby first bursts into the world, when the little fingers of their new baby wrap around your finger for the first time. Watching the kid ride a bike for the first time and passing on your knowledge and seeing them apply it and take on the world. Both spouses long for that. It's why you started trying in the first place.

You need to remember that men set up expectations for their lives as well. Michael also grew up in a family where "the family" was a focus. I wasn't there, but I know his parents and his sisters, so I'm sure the idea of him having his own family was often mentioned. I'm sure as he experienced life, both in good and bad ways, his mom taught him how he can learn from the experience and help his own children one day. He too grew up in a church where the focus of family is huge. Instead of learning how to nurture his family, like I was learning, he was learning how to stand strong and stand as an example to his children. What choices to make to help influence his family to live righteously. Without anyone being wrong, that expectation was placed on him to have children and a family, and he soon adopted that expectation on himself.

When he turned thirty he was struggling. At the time we were living in San Diego. He was at a kind of dead-end job with a boss who was a crazy control freak. There was no real plan for the future, just a bunch of ideas of what we wanted our future to be. He kind of was nowhere he thought he would be. I used to make fun of Michael, every birthday, because he gets so gloomy about his age. This year I poked fun in front of some friends as we were leaving church. This friend was old enough to be our father so had some experience behind him. He told Michael that his friend went through the same thing when they turned thirty. He told his friend to keep his head up because he had a wife, children and his own business. Then slapped Michael on the back and said, "So, see, it's not that bad." We got in the car and Michael said, "Yeah, but I don't have any of that."

I think, as a society, we forget that men plan too. Women are generally the planners, the organizers, whatever you want to call it. However, men make plans. They take their same life experiences and make and create expectations of their life. Then, just like women, when those expectations are not met, it's disappointing. It's frustrating. It causes heartache and scars. Just like it does for women.

When asking Michael what his input was on this book, this idea of infertility and how it affects him, he first mentioned that he wanted to emphasize the good that comes out of having life end up differently than what you expected. We laughed as we thought about where our life would be if we would have had our first child when we first wanted to. We laughed because it's uncomfortable to think about, because our lives would be drastically different and life seemed good where we were. He also said that it's important to know that both struggle. Men and women are different and push through their struggles differently. However, it's important to remember both sides of the couple.

Chapter 19

Through couples' struggles are disagreements about what to do for treatment, different ideas of when and how to get money, different expectations of how you are going to go about the journey. You are both so passionate about this idea and getting an end result, but are two different human beings with different upbringings so the couple must find a new way of compromising on something you may not feel you should even compromise on.

When we have considered different ideas for adoption or treatment over the years we have had some disagreements. The one that kept getting us caught was the egg donation IVF. He kept saying he wanted to pass on his DNA and I kept stopping it. I wasn't comfortable with it and his desire to pass on his DNA was not enough to sway me. It didn't happen overnight. As stated it took convincing words from a doctor and this idea that I could actually be pregnant to make me finally hear what he was saying. He still had an opportunity to pass on his DNA. Why should I be the one who stops him from that? He wasn't asking to go have a child with another woman. He was saying he wanted a child that came from him and even though that baby can't have pieces of what I look like, it could have pieces of what he looked like, and still have pieces of me. It's such a strange compromise but a real one. A real series of conversations where I shut him down over and over again; a conversation that happens in couples' bedrooms all throughout the world. It's just, yet, another way people struggle to get through it.

Here we were, though, after months of talking and me finally being on board, we were at Egg Donation IVF.

The path of egg donation IVF was yet another troubling road, however, it had seemed to be the most promising. I honestly felt like it was our last official try and I had high hopes it will work.

Egg donation IVF is, probably, the most expensive option. Not only do we have to pay for the IVF but we have to pay for the egg. I did have a young lady at one point who offered her eggs for free. She will never in this life know and understand what that did for me. That drove me to really understand the option of doing this and that really it was going to be ok. Really, it would be my baby and the DNA of this girl would run through my baby and I would have a constant reminder of the amazing thing she did for us.

It didn't work out that we were going to use her eggs; time moved forward and we are waiting to do the procedure and her life needed to move on. It was my choice to move on from using her. She didn't even really know I made it. I just didn't want her to feel obligated to anything.

With looking into egg donation I found a lot of answers to a lot of frustrations. I learned that there is an Estrogen pill I can take along with a progesterone pill that gives me the ability to cycle. It evened out my periods and my hormones and has made me feel somewhat normal again. It's amazing what a little bit of estrogen does for your body.

When I first started taking the estrogen and progesterone I started to notice a huge difference in my body. Infertility is an imbalance of hormones in your body for whatever reason. In my case it's a lack of hormones. This lack of hormones has effects I didn't notice were gone until they started to come back. I had lost a sex drive, I had lost energy and desire — desire to just like get up in the morning and live my life. It's not depression. It's just a lack of drive and push you need in order to move your life forward. Also, since I had lost a lot of these hormones, I was experiencing the ever so horrible night sweats and hot flashes. My mother-in-law explained hot flashes best, "You just want to take off your skin and run around naked." It's horrible. It's like overall you lose your livelihood. The person that you are and want to be gets lost in a lack of an ability to be you. It's harder to maintain friendships and relationships. It's harder to care about anything, including yourself. At times I felt I was trapped in a shell of a body with an idea of a person I used to want to be. It's hard to have energy to push yourself to become a better person when the hormones needed to do so just simply aren't there.

A key part of what I just talked about is the lack of sex drive. Let's talk about sex and infertility. Just sex overall loses anything it ever is or was. At some point in the process, sex goes from a great way to blow off steam, a wordless way to express love to your spouse, a deeply emotional experience that takes you and your partner away from the world and allows you to connect and be together, to something else. It takes those amazing things and turns it into a regiment that is not fun, exciting, spontaneous, or sexy. It becomes a chore. Anyone who has ever actively tried to get pregnant in their life knows the work that goes into planning sex around ovulation. You mark your calendar, count your days, pay attention to every drop of your period and every feeling in your body. Then on days you are ovulating you plan sex. The hardest part about this is everyone, doctors included, seem to have different opinions about what you should do around the day you ovulate. Some suggest having sex every day starting 2-3 days before you are supposed to ovulate for 7 days straight. Some say to only have sex during those three days you are ovulating. Some say to have sex every other day. Then, there are about

150 million things you and your spouse can do to make sure that the sperm is good and gets to the eggs. What is right?

After a few months of not getting pregnant you start to kind of do it all. You make sure the man goes nowhere near a hot tub, laptop, sauna, or anything that has been "known" to hurt the sperm. You don't even let him take a spinning class! Then, after sex you have your legs in the air, stand on your head, don't move, tilt your pelvis or anything else you can think of to help "gravity do its work."

A few months after that starts into the ovulation tests and obsessive temperature taking. Yes, you can see if you are ovulating based on your temperatures. You are supposed to temp yourself at the same time every morning. As your temperature starts to change, it is a sign that you are ovulating. After you pee on yet another expensive ovulation stick to confirm, you become on high alert and do that oh so sexy scheduled sex. You have to measure the ovulation sticks though. You keep these peed on sticks and tape them in notebooks to ensure that the line is actually getting darker so you can have sex on exactly the right day. Sounds fun and not at all stressful, right? This is why people say that you need to "stop trying" and just relax. You have no idea what stage in the trying to have a baby process that person is. They could be thousands and thousands of dollars into fertility treatments that don't work. Maybe it is true for some that relaxing is what they need but it's the smaller percentage of people. Plus, once you have it in your mind you want a child there is no turning that off. There is no stopping. What you should do is ask them if they want to talk about it. Or, if you don't really care to know, or not wanting to get into the topic, let them know you are sorry and you wish them luck.

All of these activities involved with trying to get pregnant, for me, over time, just took the joy out of sex. Then, when it turns out we weren't even getting pregnant, I started to wonder what the point even was. Why have sex at all? Isn't the idea and point of sex to procreate? The work and frustration that came with it all just paralyzed my want. It put a wedge in my marriage that I didn't expect to be put there. I had to really work through, and honestly I don't think Michael and I ever recovered from, the mental blocks that are created from "unsuccessful sex". An activity that is supposed to be fun and easy became work and overwhelming to even deal with.

Going back to egg donation IVF. I had talked to two doctors about doing the procedure and it felt pretty positive. It's still not 100%, but they felt confident, and that was a first. I also had something to look forward to. I had a plan in place instead of wandering. The concern became the size of my uterus and the thickness of my uterine lining. Without consistent periods over many years, both of these things decreased in size, and are needed in order to have a successful pregnancy.

As frustrating as everything always is in every step of this path, Michael and I had decided it would be best to put off the egg donation IVF for just a little bit longer in order to get some things in place. Unfortunately, this meant that it is too late for me to get pregnant. The size of my uterus and my uterine lining will just never be what is needed in order to have a successful pregnancy. Yet another roadblock full of regrets.

All that is left is egg donation IVF with a surrogate. I have shared a lot of personal information about my life over these pages. I have been very open in hopes that you will understand a small percentage of what a woman with infertility is going through. I hope you can understand that some things are just unexplainable. There are mental blocks and hurdles we are forced to face, no matter our trials in life, and you (all of you and me) have to find a way to get past those mental blocks. Egg donation IVF with a surrogate is my never ending mental block. Michael wants to pass on his DNA and I can't fault him for that. I can't. I don't. However, I also deserve to feel comfortable with how my child is brought into the world.

I seem crazy right? I spend all this time talking about wanting a child so bad and it seems I'm willing to do anything, so why not this? I don't know. I can't answer it. It just makes me uncomfortable. So here we are at a rock and a hard place. No right decision on either end. Leaving me at my journeys end. No feelings of ease and not ready to give up but nothing else to hold on to.

Infertility is so hard and so much is sacrificed in a person. In the end Michael and I just could not hold it together. Not just because of infertility, but just because it wasn't right. Not only were we just better as friends, we would never be able to get on the same page about how to bring a child into the world. This is important. You have to be able to agree on this in any relationship. Infertility claims the lives of marriages everywhere. We are not unique. Again, infertility wasn't why we got divorced but it was part of it.

Chapter 20

D ivorce is hard and challenging. Everyone who has gone through one knows. Sometimes the right thing feels impossible. Through all of the divorce craziness, I decided to reset my life and set sites on moving back to Idaho, where I grew up. A lot of my support system is there and I needed that support so much. How is it that when you move you find yourself surrounded by packed boxes, lists of things you still need to do and are in total and complete disarray? Because that is just what happens when you move. One really good thing about moving is that you get to go through all of your shit and decide what is garbage, what can be donated and what is actually worth moving over 1600 miles; this includes the baby stuff Michael had once packed away and we had held onto for so long. For me, right away I knew I was ready to get rid of the crib and the changing table. It's bulky and not worth moving. However, this is harder than one may think. First, I couldn't find the hardware for any of it. Second, thrift stores won't take that stuff for liability reasons. So it just sat in my house and caused insane anxiety for a good forty-eight hours. I sadly finally just threw it away. The need to get this giant, looming reminder that I am not having a baby any time soon out of my house overcame the sadness of thinking it wouldn't go to a good home.

The harder part of the baby stuff when deciding what to do with it was the two giant boxes stuffed with everything you could possibly need for a baby sitting in the top shelves of my closet. I decided I wasn't ready to let them go, and that was ok. But then one night while lying in my bed I was counting boxes because the moving company needed to know how many I had, and thinking about those two boxes they suddenly became nuisances. It was in that moment that I decided I was ready to let them go — let go of my hope that a bouncing baby boy was going to show up in my house any time soon.

I have a friend that is just starting out in her life. She just got married and moved far away from home and her whole life is ahead of her. Even though she does not want a baby right now she does eventually. While talking to her one morning it dawned on me that I should give the baby stuff to her! And she wanted it! I was so excited I pulled down the boxes to rip them open and show her what was inside. The moment I ripped open the first box it was as if time froze. I was suddenly looking at a very dark part of my past and an equally dark part of my present. Once the moment passed I started to pull stuff out. It was like going through ghosts of the past. Each little blanket and onesie and sock and book was a deep and sharp reminder that this adoption never happened. My baby never came. Not only that, but I am getting a divorce. I am not only not closer to getting a baby, but I am now even further away. As I lovingly went through these items, I realized that this was the very first time I had looked through any of this since they had been packed up. Some of them even still smelled like a baby. I cried a lot. Tears fell for everything. Everything that has happened since I thought I would be getting a child.

It was in this moment that I was reminded that life is never what you think it will be. It's always harder and sometimes appears to never get easier. I am here to tell you with firm understanding that it's never easy to "just adopt". The cost and emotions that come with it are astronomical. I don't know if I will ever heal from my wounds. I don't know if I will ever have the courage again to try and adopt. Pains from my past are still here in my heart in the present. For now, I decided while going through the stuff that I will just keep that fox that sat in Atticus's crib. Yeah, he had a name – Atticus William – strong name. This fox will be in my house as a reminder that it's okay to be sad about the loss of a child I never had and was never mine to begin with. A reminder of a marriage that was. A reminder that I can move on and life does create silver linings in every hardship. A reminder that I will be okay.

Being okay meant a lot of different things for me. Moving home to Idaho was hands down the best idea I have ever had in my life. Being close to family and friends and in a place that was so much of who I am helped me reset and rediscover me. That doesn't mean the transition was easy. I struggled. About a month after moving home and living alone for the second time in my life — but really more like the first, because the first time I was in high school— COVID hit. I sat alone in my apartment with COVID for 2 weeks. It. Was. Horrible. I did have things that connected me to people, but I was so lonely. Everything felt so unsure.

Chapter 21

A round this time, I started online dating again. Online dating sucks. Well, dating sucks, we all know it. Adding to it that, everything is closed, no one is supposed to be in contact, and that makes it harder. I would talk to people over text or calls but nothing really stuck. I did meet up with a guy and we casually dated for about a month, but it didn't go anywhere. I remember the night we broke up. My friends and I were at a cabin in Island Park. Even though I knew this guy was not the one for me it still wasn't a great experience, and I wanted an outlet. After some drinking, we all started talking about dating apps, Tinder specifically. I said I felt that pretty much it's paid prostitution since you have to pay for the app, but the woman never gets the money. Keep in mind I was drunk and knew nothing of the app. That's when one friend's fifteen-year-old said that actually you don't have to pay. How he knew that I will never know but beyond the point. So, we felt, naturally, that we needed to investigate. That's how I joined Tinder. Why is there shame in that sentence? That night we all drunkenly swiped left on a bunch of guys that you just knew were waiting to send you some nasty dick pics. It was actually a great source of entertainment for a lot of us. What I found, though, is that there was actually some cute and decent looking guys in there and maybe worth swiping right on. I thought to myself, why not?

I will make a long story short and mention a few things I really learned about dating and how my Tinder experience ended. First, I felt the need to be upfront about my inability to have children. I don't want to put myself in a situation where I fall in love with someone and then tell them I can't have children and land back at square one because they too have a deep need to pass on their DNA. So, when do you tell them? How do you tell them? There is no good answer if you are looking for one. Two, you learn that a lot of men who are in their 30's and don't have kids, because they don't want kids at all. How do you approach this? I felt like I was in this weird situation where either I am forced to date a guy with kids, wasn't sure how I felt about that yet, or date a guy who didn't want kids. Again, I don't know the solution to these problems. I just know the problem I was in. Since I was newly out of a marriage and my one-month guy I dated didn't go great I felt that just casual dating was going to be my scene. A guy I had met and talked to on Tinder, Robert, seemed like a perfect fit. That's what Tinder is, right? Casual…

Robert was recently divorced, like even more recent than me. He had married his high school sweetheart and they were together for a total of about thirteen years. I will never forget the first time I saw him in person. I pulled up next to his big blue truck in the Jamba Juice parking lot and he hopped out. He came around his hood and smiled at me. I thought, "Holy shit, he is actually really cute." We spent our first date sipping smoothies and walking around the Greenbelt in Idaho Falls. We talked about a lot. It was a very easy first date. First date led to several more dates and getting to know each other at a more personal level. Through getting to know each other, with no walls up or guards — I mean we were just casually dating — Robert and I somehow ended up getting really serious. I assume the no walls or guards thing. We found ourselves spending every free moment we had with each other and falling in love.

I learned that Robert and his ex wife had decided to not have children. He did, though, have two nephews that idolized him. "Uncle D" was very involved in their lives and I noticed a fatherly role he took with them. These boys do have a pretty awesome dad but Robert took on a role stronger than a typical uncle. I saw how much he cared for them and how much they appreciated the love of an uncle who really cared.

Naturally, as we became more and more serious the talk of families came up. I was never concerned about Robert actually wanting children, because of the way he interacted with his nephews. However, we did have to have some conversations to really make sure we were on the same page. What I learned is that it was his ex wife who really didn't want kids. Robert was okay with the idea of not having kids, but was never really anti-kids. Our conversations gave him a different outlook. He now had a different partner that did want children. Knowing this, he could picture a future with a kid or two, and was happy with what that meant for our road ahead. After I really understood his past and why he didn't have kids, I realized that I was with a partner whose love was so unconditional that no matter our future ahead; our own kids, adopted kids, puppies, he would be happy and we would be happy together.

Robert and I now own a house and are really looking forward to our life together. We happened to enter each other's lives at the worst and best time. Our casual idea turned into a deep connection that we later named magnetism and somehow ended up here. With this something happened in me. I have heard of this phenomenon before but never thought I would experience it and given my situation and history didn't think it would come up. Here I am with this guy who I love and want to spend the rest of my life with. What does that mean? I want a family with him.

Before our first date I told Robert I couldn't have kids. I told him that was a weird thing to say before we even went on a date, but I felt he needed to know. He told me that it was okay, and due to some experiences in his life he recognized that parenthood doesn't always come in the form of DNA, then said that maybe we can talk about family planning after the first date. We laughed. That being said, I still want a family with this man.

I found myself kind of at the beginning again. This, like, weird feeling of "this could actually happen" got dusted off and brought to the surface. It was confusing and hurtful. It had been so long since Michael and I were in a good place, that being in this happy relationship with someone who I loved and loved me so much gave me feelings of hope I thought I had gotten rid of. In the first five or six months of dating Robert I took two pregnancy tests. One was like an old-fashioned way of Robert knowing it was happening and we both wondering and worrying what the result would be, bringing a reality of what we weren't prepared for to the forefront. The second was old school Luanne. Where I was out of town and it was that cycle of self-hatred and instant regret mixed with depression. On top of this pregnancy cycle depression came just feelings of regret. Regret for so many things in my life related to infertility. Also regret, and some disappointment in myself, that I had allowed myself to feel like this again.

That is so funny to think about. How can we be so angry at ourselves for feelings — feelings that are real and justified? Yet here I was just mad. Confused. Unsure. I had somehow created narratives in my head that it might work with Robert. That things might be different. How would it be different though? Michael was not the problem. I had no eggs. I even went to the gynecologist and had them do a check to make sure my medications were set right. But this feeling of expecting a miracle had bubbled up and I had no idea how to control it.

In 2020, while dealing with COVID and all hell that it brought, I was having some major health problems. My blood sugar was struggling, and I pretty much had a UTI from May until December, and no one could quite figure out what was happening. A friend of mine recommended a doctor's office in town that was well known for their homeopathic approach on medicine mixed with modern medicine. She said she had heard amazing results from people of this doctor helping with problems that other doctors couldn't seem to figure out the solution to. On their website, after looking into them, I saw that their approach is fixing the problem, not treating the symptom. I decided to give it a shot.

My first appointment there I spent about a half hour telling the doctor everything that was wrong with me. I did include the information about the random period I had that year without prompt and struggles I had been having with the estrogen I normally took. He was a gynecologist by trade and known for his miracles with people being able to have babies so I assumed he could figure out what was going on with my hormones along with my UTIs.

After a half hour of talking, he addressed my issues and said what he thought would help the blood sugars and the UTIs. Then said what a lot of doctors like to say. That I was young and he was disappointed to see that I had seemed to have given up on having children. He recommended that we look into it and see what he could find. He said he made no promises but recommended I watch a video they had on their website of a miracle he had recently seen in a woman they had treated.

I told Robert everything the doctor had said. Robert, being a level-headed guy, reminded me that I should focus on getting healthy and not put a lot of hope into the other part. I knew he was right. I was already thinking this and had committed myself to not get my hopes up for anything. There were two weeks before my next appointment. I tried with everything I had to not get any hopes up. Little did I realize that inside I had hoped that this was it. This would be the time one doctor, out of many, was right. He could perform the miracle and we would be blessed with one.

Two weeks went by and I was back in his office. We found easy solutions to the blood sugar and UTI problem and I was quite relieved to know that nightmare would be over. Then he said, now about the hormones… I suddenly felt very old feelings and very old coping mechanisms pop up. I sat up and put on this weird smile I only have in this situation. I had the old feeling of realizing I was in this room alone. Yes, a doctor was there but no one there to hold my hand. I had suddenly wished I had invited RD to come with me. I know he would have. The doctor told me what doctors had told me for years, nothing had changed. I still could not have kids and no treatment was going to help. There was one very experimental treatment and he had no idea if it would work or not. I had that to think about and was sent on my way. As I walked to the checkout and to my car I felt that old feeling of holding in any emotion or reaction to the news. I just had to get to my car.

I didn't want to tell Robert over the phone. However, I had the app Marco Polo and two best friends on the other side. I told them everything the doctor said and sobbed. Why was I sobbing? In the moment I didn't know. I just knew that once again here I was. I was in this state of despair, grief, unsure of my future and frankly just not knowing what to do. It would be hours before Robert got home and I spent most of that time in this depressed state. I cried so much and just laid on my couch with a blanket in despair. Since I am a writer I decided to write what I was feeling and this is what I said:

"I don't know what I am feeling right now. Sad and defeated is the only words that come to mind. The thing is today a new option was given to me. You would think I would feel a level of excitement. Even a small percentage presented. So why do I feel so sad? Maybe because it wasn't a great option. Maybe because it was so expensive. I don't know. Why am I sad? I felt myself sitting there. I felt the same emotions I had before. I felt that weird brave smile I have that only exists in this situation. It's like a mask that envelopes my face. I am feeling old emotions right now. Emotion I was past, I thought. Emotion that has been buried deep. I don't know if I want to revisit this. Maybe I just want to move on. Obviously, though, I don't move on. What do I do? How do I get past this? How do I move on? Maybe I don't. I know sometimes you have to try every avenue until you have moved on. Did I not feel every avenue was visited? Do I feel I look down a road and see a dead end? Do I not know enough? I am realizing that I saw hope. Then I saw the same look on every doctor's face I have ever seen. I heard the reaction I hear every time. I then feel alone. I was alone in this room all over again. I was isolated from my feelings. Hope hides. It hides in dark places. It masks itself. It pretends it's not there. I hate hope."

I left my computer open and started dinner. Robert and I talked and talked and talked and talked. I cried so much. I was confused and unsure.

The next morning I woke up unsure of what to do. How to approach the situation. After getting ready, I came to my desk to work and saw my personal computer was still open. I decided to reread what I had written the night before. As I was reading, I read the words of someone who is trapped — trapped in this idea that some day the perfect situation may present itself and I will get pregnant. I felt bad for her. I stared at the words I had written and thought about a lot Robert and I had talked about. In that moment, I realized I was done. Done with this cycle. The small amount of hope I had allowed myself mixed with an experimental treatment that was a lot of money and offered zero guarantees sparked these feelings of confusion. I was so over feeling them that mixed in with feelings of defeat from the doctors words were feelings of being over feeling the feelings I had. I don't want to be down this road anymore. I hate it. I hate the ups and downs I have faced. I hate the tears I have cried alone, I hate the sadness of each failed step. I am over it. Over it. I then, in that moment, let go of all of it. I decided I was officially done trying to get pregnant and hoping I ever would.

Chapter 22

Since that moment my life has been different. For one, I was able to reread and finish my book in order to get passed off to an editor and give hope one day it may be published. I finally felt my story is over. Adoption will be in my future when Robert and I feel we are at the step of children. Also, a new baby is in my life right now. I have been able to look at him different and appreciate his milestones differently than I have with other babies in the past. I have seen pregnancy announcements and have felt instant excitement and very little pings of jealousy, even though they are there. I finally look at my life ahead and accept it may or may not have children. I finally realize that really and truly when it comes to this terrible unseen disease of infertility, my journey has ended.

Of course, the journey is never over. I will always grieve. I will always wish. I will always want.

The question was once asked to me. What is it about not having my own children that I am unwilling to leave behind. What brings me the most sadness when thinking about it? I had to really think about it. I imagine this answer is different for most people. For me, I realized, it's the idea of not passing on my DNA is what I grasped onto and can't seem to leave behind.

I hate my double chin, tire belly, hairy toes, and thick black hair that grows on my legs. However, I know exactly where those attributes come from. My feet were so bad that I had to get surgery on one in order to walk and run. This surgery was terrible and the recovery took way longer than I ever wanted. However, I know exactly where those bad feet came from. On the better side, my cute nose that makes for a great profile, my long fingers that help me play piano, and my thick hair on my head that is my pride and joy all bring me happiness. I know where those attributes came from. I love that when I stand next to my dad I look just like him. I love that when I'm next to my mom everyone knows we belong together. I love that when we stand as a family...or I guess I should say stood as a family... I was the one that looked like both parents, and so it looked like I brought us together. I helped make us look like a family. I know that behaviors are learned, but DNA is who we are. I don't get to pass on who I am. My kids don't get to have my long fingers. They don't get my long, thick hair. Their nose will never look like mine. When we go to the doctor and give family medical history mine will never be included. I will not physically be in my child, ever.

I know what you are thinking. That I will pass onto my children other things. However, I ask you what do you think connects you to your child most? How do you know without a doubt that child is yours? Is it the way he scrunches his nose just like you do? Is the way she stands and holds up her finger and sasses you like you are looking in a tiny mirror? I will never have that. I am just afraid I will never hold that ultimate connection that connects parent to child.

I know someone who did sperm donation with her ex-husband. The divorce didn't leave them friends and apparently he won't ever win as dad of the year. She told me once that he wasn't actually her dad and didn't even deserve to see her. I'm not arguing that he maybe didn't deserve time spent with her based on his actions (I know little of the story). What I am saying is that there are people in the world; people I may add that I know and love, who have this mindset; who think that what defines a child is a blood relation. So what does that make me? How do I fit in? I don't ever get to be the real mom. Just a substitute.

That the hole in my heart, my soul, that is supposed to be filled by a child still remains gaping and yearning to be filled will most likely never be. The sadness, even though I have accepted it will always be there to haunt me in moments.

As I look in my past I see my bad days. They caught me by surprise what would trigger me. Sometimes it was a holiday, like fucking Mother's Day. Sometimes it was a movie where the feelings of the movie echoed my feelings of loss. Sometimes it was a TV show where someone has a baby and I wondered if I ever will. Whatever it was, I used to become so depressed I couldn't even move. I would lay on the bed or on the couch and just do nothing but stare at the TV. I sobbed pretty uncontrollably off and on. I tried to snap out of it. I tried to do things to distract me but I couldn't even move. I was paralyzed in sadness. It's different from other bad days. When it's sadness about infertility, there's nothing I could say or do. I knew I had been blessed and I had great things in my life but there is nothing I could say to myself because I couldn't see the future. I couldn't see if I was going to have a child and if the hole in my heart would ever be filled. If I would ever have what I have been planning for, yearning for, and expecting in my life. I didn't know if all of those fun traditions I had with my family as a child will be able to be passed on. I didn't know if I will ever see my partner holding a teeny little baby with love in his eyes that fathers only have for their children.

One of the worst things about these days is I didn't know who to talk to about it. I didn't want to talk to my friends or family because it's the same story over and over again. It's the same words and thoughts and feelings and nothing ever changes. Wouldn't they be sick of that? During one of my bad days I did message some friends saying what I was feeling. I debated hitting send just because I knew there was nothing they could do or say and I knew they knew that. I told them I should just shut up about it, so they knew they didn't have to respond. I then sent it. My friend messaged back and said, "You don't have to shut up. I'm sorry you have to go through that, Lu." Turns out it was exactly what I needed to hear. As a friend that's all you ever need to say — validate the feelings and remind me that I have a reason to be sad and it's ok. When this friend said those things this particular time, I did start crying immediately and cried for a good ten minutes. I curled up in a ball and just waited for it to pass. There was something about giving myself permission to be sad about it because my friend said I could be that gave me the ability to really cry about it. Then, I was able to slowly come out of it and ended the day ok. I don't always have the ability to be ok to talk about it yet somehow I always find a way to push through, pull myself together and move past the sadness.

Even as I read through that now I remember those hard days and struggles on holidays and I feel sad for me, for what I have gone through. My sadness surrounding infertility will never end. I will always be envious of others and wish their fertility on me. However, those bad days are behind me. Even if I do feel sad about it from time to time I am not paralyzed or overcome with so much sadness I don't know what to do with it. Then in these moments I know I can turn to Robert and will listen, love and comfort.

Over the years I have learned so much. I have learned a lot about myself, about other women and about what it's truly like to struggle. Mainly, what I have learned is that infertility is a quiet struggle. It mostly exists in your mind and the horrible thoughts and heart wrenching fears just stay locked up spinning and swirling in your head sometimes non-stop and sometimes very loud. It often feels so lonely.

Because of infertility I have experienced a lot of heartache. I have felt sadness like you wouldn't believe and loneliness that is emptier than any loss I have ever had.

However, because of infertility I have lived. I know I will be ok. I know that I am ok. I can look through life, see all the opportunities I have had and what amazing experiences I have experienced, people I've met and adventures I have been on. I can look through and see that the blessings I get from not being able to have children are astronomical. Of course I would want to have children but I can't focus on that all the time. I can allow myself to go through my bad days, hard feelings and struggles but as I start to come out of those and want to feel happy with my life I can look and see how I have been blessed even without children.

When you first started reading this I know you thought the same thing that people have told me over and over again as I introduced them to the beginning of my book. You read that opener and thought, "Infertility does not define you." I am here to tell you it has. It has made me strong, it has made me understanding, it has made me patient. It has taught me to focus on the good in my life. It has given me an amazing career and career path. It has given me strength. It has made me who I am today. I am proud to be infertile. I am proud to stand up and say I can't have kids and it equally sucks and is ok. Being grateful for a trial is impossible at times but we have to be. We have to be grateful for what we have in life. We have to be grateful for lessons learned. If we don't we only ever see the bad and finding the joy in life will be impossible.

To the women out there who are also infertile:

Whether you have one hundred babies or none, if you want another and can't have one, it's okay to be sad. It's okay to cry. It's okay to be scared and frustrated and mad. It's okay to not feel proud. It's okay to not feel grateful. The only thing that is not okay is to feel alone. Okay, you can feel alone, but you have to pull out of that feeling. It's hard. It's hard to not feel alone but you are not. You are not alone at all. There are thousands of women and families struggling just like you. Their struggle may look different. Just remember, though, they are just as scared as you are. They are just as lost as you are. And they feel just as poor as you do. We are in this together and create a silent bond that is stronger than you know. We are here to hold your hand and hear you cry. We will cry together when times are tough and rejoice together when we have any sort of success.

As you struggle in sadness, just remember how the elephant replies to the dog when the dog asks why it has had litters of puppies several times in the two years the elephant has taken to grow one baby. "There is something I want you to understand. What I am carrying is not a puppy, but an elephant. I can only give birth to one in two years. When my baby hits the ground, the earth feels it. When my baby crosses the road, human beings stop and watch in admiration. What I carry draws attention. So, what I'm carrying is mighty and great - and takes time."

What you are waiting for and what you are making is amazing. I wish and hope it is a baby one day. For those who may never have one know that your story and your life is just as amazing. What you are making and creating for the world is just as impactful as this baby elephant. It's ok to be defined by infertility but don't let it cripple you. Stand tall. Be your own elephant and never give up hope. Whatever hope may mean.